The
Stress Free
Diabetes Kitchen

Over 140 easy & delicious diabetes recipes
designed for no-hassle cooking

by Barbara Seelig-Brown

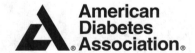

American
Diabetes
Association®

Director, Book Publishing, Abe Ogden; Managing Editor, Greg Guthrie; Acquisitions Editor, Victor Van Beuren; Editor, Rebekah Renshaw; Production Manager, Melissa Sprott; Composition, ADA; Cover Design, Vis-á-Vis Creative Concepts; Photographer, Renee Comet; Printer, United Graphics, Inc.

Printed in the United States of America

1 3 5 7 9 10 8 6 4 2

The suggestions and information contained in this publication are generally consistent with the Clinical Practice Recommendations and other policies of the American Diabetes Association, but they do not represent the policy or position of the Association or any of its boards or committees. Reasonable steps have been taken to ensure the accuracy of the information presented. However, the American Diabetes Association cannot ensure the safety or efficacy of any product or service described in this publication. Individuals are advised to consult a physician or other appropriate health care professional before undertaking any diet or exercise program or taking any medication referred to in this publication. Professionals must use and apply their own professional judgment, experience, and training and should not rely solely on the information contained in this publication before prescribing any diet, exercise, or medication. The American Diabetes Association—its officers, directors, employees, volunteers, and members—assumes no responsibility or liability for personal or other injury, loss, or damage that may result from the suggestions or information in this publication.

☺ The paper in this publication meets the requirements of the ANSI Standard Z39.48-1992 (permanence of paper). ADA titles may be purchased for business or promotional use or for special sales. To purchase more than 50 copies of this book at a discount, or for custom editions of this book with your logo, contact the American Diabetes Association at the address below, at booksales@diabetes.org, or by calling 703-299-2046.

American Diabetes Association
1701 North Beauregard Street
Alexandria, Virginia 22311

DOI: 10.2337/9781580404600

Library of Congress Cataloging-in-Publication Data
Seelig-Brown, Barbara.
 The stress-free diabetes kitchen : over 140 easy and delicious diabetes recipes designed for no-hassle cooking / Barbara Seelig-Brown.
     p. cm.
  Summary: "This book will help the reader establish a useful pantry, fridge, and freezer. These "staples" will allow the reader pull out this book and cook just about anything, in a stress-free way"-- Provided by publisher.
 Includes bibliographical references and index.
 ISBN 978-1-58040-460-0 (pbk.)
 1. Diabetes--Diet therapy--Recipes. I. Title.
 RC662.S448 2012
 641.5'6314--dc23
                    2012003340

Contents

Acknowledgments

DEDICATION: For Barone with never ending love. You were the dream husband who helped me accomplish my dream. I wouldn't have been able to publish even one cookbook without your love, encouragement, tasting skills, and wine expertise. If only I could cook for you one more time. Thank you to all those who made this book possible with your encouragement and support:

To Laurie and Val Burzynski, our dream friends, for sharing some of Ma's recipes, the tried and true Italian family favorites are exactly what I look for in a great meal. When Al and I called you our dream friends, no one knew what that would mean. You live it everyday.

To my mother, who taught me the value of home cooking.

To my family, who allow me the joy of cooking for them.

To the staff at the ADA: Rebekah Renshaw, for her generous editing and patience; Abe Ogden, for considering this idea; and to Heschel Falek, for marketing *The Diabetes Seafood Cookbook* in a way that made this book possible. Thanks also to Lyn Wheeler who did the nutrition analysis for the recipes, as well as Renee Comet for the beautiful photography and Lisa Cherkasky and Carolyn Schimley for the food styling.

Thank you all with love and appreciation,

Barbara Seelig-Brown

CHAPTER 1:
The Stress Free Pantry

The Stress Free Diabetes Kitchen

What is Stress Free Cooking?

I love being the Stress Free Cook because it's a great conversation starter. I love to cook. Even if you don't like to cook, most of you might <u>have</u> to cook at one time or another. Cooking at home makes us more in control of what and how we eat.

If you are reading this, you care about what you put into your body. When I work with kids, I tell them to think of their body as a Ferrari. You would only put the best fuel in your Ferrari, so you should do the same for your body. Learning about food and nutrition is the best way to know what fuel you should put into your body. One of the easiest ways to begin the journey to good nutrition is by simply thinking of using color on the plate. Preparing a meal with color is like taking a Nutrition 101 class without hitting the books. Since we eat with our eyes, it also makes any plate more appealing to us.

Another way to have a Stress Free Kitchen is to gather a dependable repertoire of versatile recipes that become your "go to" recipes. The kind of recipes that you love and can make with your eyes closed. I hope you will find those recipes in this book. Make copies of them and keep them in your kitchen cupboard so you will have them at your fingertips. Soon, making them will become second nature to you. Feel free to mix and match the sauces, marinades, dressings, and side dishes in this book. My recipes are all about versatility and you will find serving suggestions and tips to help you.

I also provide you with a list of items to keep in your pantry, fridge, and freezer. These "staples" will allow you pull out this book and cook just about anything you are in the mood for. I want you to spend more time in your kitchen cooking instead of wasting valuable cooking time running to the market. I would much rather be home in my bunny slippers, cooking a great meal, as opposed to standing in a grocery store or take-out line. I've also included a list of equipment that you should have in your kitchen at all times.

Essential Pantry List

PANTRY STAPLES

Extra virgin olive oil

Balsamic, white balsamic, and wine vinegars

Sea salt—fine grind

Garlic—fresh, whole heads

Onions

Shallots

Pepper corns and a good quality pepper mill

Flour—all purpose, white wheat, Wondra (granulated flour that is very light and absorbs less oil)

Yeast

Honey

Sugar—white, brown, and a natural sugar substitute

Pasta—whole grain and regular in a variety of shapes and sizes

Rice—jasmine, arborio (for risotto)

Beans (canned)—black beans, pink beans, chickpeas, small white beans

Lentils—small green, brown, and red

Polenta/corn meal

Evaporated skim milk

Low-sodium canned broth and stock—chicken, beef, mushroom, vegetable

Low-sodium diced tomatoes, crushed tomatoes, tomato paste

Fruits (canned)—Mandarin oranges, apricots, crushed pineapple

Fruits (dried)—raisins, cherries, apricots

REFRIGERATOR

Low-fat cottage cheese

Part skim ricotta cheese

Crumbled low-fat gorgonzola

Low-fat, plain yogurt

Fresh mozzarella

High-Quality, full flavor cheeses, such as Parmigiano-Reggiano, Grana Padano, and Asiago

Eggs—large

Mustard—variety

Capers

Wine—dry white

Lemons

Limes

Oranges

Salad greens—a variety of types, textures, and colors

Fresh baby spinach

Carrots

Celery

Fresh herbs—basil, oregano, rosemary

Sun-dried tomatoes (found in produce section, not in oil)

Olives

FREEZER

Filled pastas—tortellini, agnolotti

Phyllo

Homemade bread crumbs

Artichokes

Baby corn

Peas

String beans—whole

Pearl onions

Ground beef and/or buffalo

Turkey cuts—ground, breast, thin-sliced breast for scaloppini, sausage

Chicken breasts, boneless and skinless, individually wrapped

Roasting chickens, 5–6 pound, washed and then frozen

Cornish hens

Large shrimp, cooked, peeled, and deveined

Large shrimp, uncooked, peeled, and deveined

Individually frozen fish fillets

Individually frozen center-cut pork chops

Blueberries

Raspberries

Strawberries

Pignoli nuts (pine nuts)

Crepes

ADDITIONAL ITEMS

Anything you love to cook with that fits into your meal plan. By keeping these items in stock in your kitchen you will be able to come home from a busy day and put together a colorful, delicious meal in no time using the recipes found in *The Stress Free Kitchen*.

Basic Equipment List For Stress Free Cooking

» Dough or bench scraper—to scrape pizza dough from counter

» Egg slicer—to slice eggs, olives, or strawberries

» Flat meat pounder—to pound meat into an even thickness that allows for thorough cooking. It does not pierce the meat

» Food processor—for shredding cheese, slicing veggies, and making pizza dough

» Graduated sets of mixing bowls in glass or stainless steel

» Grater/zester (such as Microplane)—for finely zested citrus or grated cheese

» Half sheet pans for baking and roasting veggies

» Immersion blender—for quick purees right in the pot

» Instant read meat thermometer—never overcook anything again

» Mis En Place dishes (see Tips for Mis En Place)

» Parchment paper—alleviates need for additional fat in pan and makes clean up easier

» Pizza stone

» Pizza cutter (pizza wheel)

» Salad spinner—greens last longer when stored with less water

» Stand mixer

» Tongs for turning meat and tossing salad

» Knives: chef's knife, paring knife, slicing knife, and serrated knife (for soft foods such as bread and tomatoes)

» Pans: 8-, 10-, 12-inch sauté or fry pans, both nonstick and traditional finish; Sauteuse pan (looks like a sauté pan but has 2 loop handles and goes conveniently into the oven); grill pan; 3- and 4- quart sauce pans, and 8- quart stock or soup pot

Tips For A Stress Free Kitchen

» Read recipes thoroughly before beginning to cook.

» Make sure you understand all the ingredients and cooking terms.

» Prepare what is referred to as Mis en place. It means that you gather all the ingredients, do all the prep such as washing, measuring, slicing, dicing, and have everything ready before turning on the stove, mixer, or food processor.

» When preparing pizza dough or yeast bread use your meat thermometer to make sure that that the water or milk is at the proper temperature, which is between 110–120 degrees.

» A good rising place is your oven, turned off, but with the oven light on. It is warm and draft free.

» Drain and rinse anything from a can. You will remove as much of any potential preservatives or flavorings that could influence your dish.

» Draining canned beans helps to remove any preservatives and some of the gas.

» Purchase the highest quality cheeses that you can for more flavor. You will be able to use less and save calories.

» Stock your kitchen with helpful tools (See Basic Equipment List, page 5).

» Microplane for grating cheese, garlic, nutmeg, chocolate and zesting citrus

» A flat meat pounder for pounding meat or chopping nuts in plastic bags

» Toast nuts by placing in a small dry skillet and cooking until golden. Remove from pan and cool. Place in plastic bag and roughly chop with your meat pounder.

» Convection oven—If your oven has a convection setting, use it to save time. You can figure that your dishes will cook in about 25% less time. Since convection ovens have a fan that evenly circulates heat, you will have more even browning as well.

» Keep extra stock or broth on hand. This will help you in a pinch such as a pan needing to be deglazed, a soup that needs a little more flavor or liquid, a sauce that needs a boost and much more. Purchase stock is large quantities and store for use all week. It will keep up to 10 days once opened.

» Deglazing is a technique that lifts the browned bits from the bottom of the pan after sautéing, browning, or searing. Simply add some liquid such as wine, stock or water to the hot pan and the bits will be released creating a more flavorful sauce.

» Crush and peel garlic with a chef's knife using this method: Place one clove of garlic on a cutting board. Place the flat side of a chef's knife on top of the garlic. With your other hand, give the chef's knife a good strong whack over the garlic. Lift up the knife and remove the papery garlic skin. The garlic is partially chopped. Continue chopping with a rocking motion until you have desired size.

» Salad Tips: Salad should not be swimming in dressing. It's better to add less and decide you need more. Drying your greens in a salad spinner will help dressing cling to the greens rather than sinking to the bottom of the salad bowl. Slowly whisking in the oil allows for a better emulsion.

» The drier your greens are when storing them, the longer they will last. Wash them, spin them dry, lay them on paper towels, roll up, and place in a plastic bag.

» Signature Herb Blend: Go through your herbs and spices and create your own "signature blend" that will be a shortcut way to season anything you are cooking. For instance, if you frequently use basil, parsley, and rosemary, go ahead and pre-mix them, add salt and pepper if desired and you have your own signature herb blend ready to use.

» Wondra is a great addition to the pantry. It is granulated flour that makes smooth sauces and also is good for searing and sautéing as it is finer and lighter than all-purpose flour and will absorb less oil.

» Place leftover artisan or homemade breads in your food processor to create your own breadcrumbs and freeze them.

» Plan meals ahead so that you can properly defrost ingredients, and know that you have everything on hand.

» Remember to cook pasta in at least 4–6 quarts of water. Cooking pasta in too small a pot or too little water will result in sticky, gummy pasta. Using a larger pot than you think you will need is a good idea.

» Easy asparagus trimming; just hold it in both hands and bend. The ends will naturally break off at the correct place.

» Keep your knives sharp—they will make your work go more quickly

» Use a large bowl or pan than you think you will need so that you don't have to switch during the cooking process and have an additional item to wash.

» Make enough salad dressing to last several days.

» Use a crockpot to cook soups, stews, and sauces while you are out.

» If the recipes calls for fresh herbs and you have only dried, you can convert dry to fresh with this ratio;
1 part dry = 3 parts fresh.

» Edible Flowers include Nasturtiums, Pansies, Roses, Marigolds, Hibiscus, and Herb flowers.

» A vegetable steamer is handy but if you don't have one, simply place the veggies in a pan with a tight fitting lid, add an inch or two of water and cook 5–10 minutes until tender. Make sure you don't let the water evaporate completely so you might want to watch this pan closely.

» To butterfly a piece of meat such as a pork tenderloin or boneless turkey breast, place the meat on the flat work surface. Find the horizontal center and cut one third of the way into the meat so that you can unfold it to one side. Repeat with other side and open the meat so that it is flat.

» Keep a permanent magic marker in your kitchen so that you can date items once opened and you won't throw out as much "questionable" food.

» Asian long beans may be difficult to find if you do not have an Asian market available. Green beans can be substituted, but their preparation will be different as they have a different cooking characteristic. Asian long beans will not steam properly. Boiling is the only way to get them to the appropriate tenderness. Regular green beans can be steamed if you prefer that method. Either bean should be boiled to the point that they have lost their crispness, but are still somewhat firm and not fully cooked (See recipe for Val's Long Bean Pasta, page 128).

Stir-Fry Guidelines

» Make sure all knives are sharp

» Do all prep (cleaning, chopping) in advance, cut longer cooking vegetables into smaller pieces than quicker cooking items.

» Partially freeze meat, fish, or chicken to make slicing easier

» Marinate meat for 1–2 hours or fish for 20 minutes.

» Assemble all ingredients in a mis en place (see Tips).

» Heat wok or large sauté pan prior to adding oil and food.

» Add oil.

» Add foods in order of cooking time—slow cooking first, then fast cooking. Cook vegetables first, remove, then cook meat or fish.

» Add seasonings and combine meat, fish, and vegetables.

» Sauces can be thickened by adding a mixture of liquid thickened with cornstarch. Basic recipe: 1 teaspoon cornstarch dissolved in 1/4 cup water or stock. Cook until sauce is thickened and clear.

CHAPTER 2:
Appetizers & Light Bites

The Stress Free Diabetes Kitchen

Appetizers & Light Bites

Basil Cups with Roasted Red Pepper and Fresh Mozzarella

SERVES: 36 / SERVING SIZE: 1 PIECE

This appetizer/hors d'oeuvre is easy to prepare, colorful, and can be made early in the day.

» 1/2 pound part skim mozzarella, cut into 36 pieces, 1-inch square and 1/8-inch thick
» 1 bunch fresh basil, washed and dried (large leaves are best)
» 4 roasted red peppers, cut into pieces slightly larger than the mozzarella
» Freshly ground pepper

1. Layer a basil leaf, a piece of roasted red pepper, and a piece of mozzarella.

2. Sprinkle freshly ground pepper on top.

3. Cover and refrigerate until serving time.

VARIATION:
Top with a rolled anchovy or capers.

Exchanges/Choices		
Free food	Calories 20	Potassium 45 mg
	Calories from Fat 10	Total Carbohydrate 1 g
	Total Fat 1.0 g	Dietary Fiber 0 g
	Saturated Fat 0.6 g	Sugars 1 g
	Trans Fat 0.0 g	Protein 2 g
	Cholesterol 5 mg	Phosphorus 35 mg
	Sodium 40 mg	

Bruschetta

Bruschetta comes from the Italian term "bruscare," which refers to bread being roasted over coals. Traditionally, Bruschetta is bread rubbed with garlic and drizzled with olive oil, salt, and pepper. In this country, we mistakenly think of Bruschetta as the chopped tomato mixture that goes on top the bruschetta. The great thing about Bruschetta is that you can top it with anything you like.

» 1 loaf Italian bread, sliced 1/2 inch on the diagonal
» Large garlic cloves, cut in half vertically.
» Extra virgin olive oil spray

1. Rub one side of the bread with the cut side of a garlic clove. Spray each slice of bread with olive oil spray. Place oiled side of bread down on grill or oiled side up under broiler. Grill or broil until golden brown.

COOK'S TIP:
Can be made a day ahead of time and placed in a plastic bag.

Exchanges/Choices
1/2 Starch
1/2 Fat

Calories 60
  Calories from Fat 15
Total Fat 1.5 g
  Saturated Fat 0.3 g
  Trans Fat 0.0 g
Cholesterol 0 mg
Sodium 110 mg

Potassium 20 mg
Total Carbohydrate 9 g
  Dietary Fiber 1 g
  Sugars 1 g
Protein 2 g
Phosphorus 20 mg

Fresh Tomato & Basil Sauce

SERVES: 8 / SERVING SIZE: 1/8 RECIPE

This no-cook sauce is great as a Bruschetta topping, a pasta sauce, or a "salsa" for a sautéed or grilled protein.

» 12 plum tomatoes, chopped
» 2 cloves garlic, minced
» 1 shallot, minced
» 2 teaspoons extra virgin olive oil
» 1 teaspoon red wine vinegar
» 1/2 teaspoon fine sea salt
» Freshly ground pepper
» 1 cup fresh basil leaves

1. Mix tomatoes, garlic, and shallot. Add olive oil, vinegar, salt, and pepper.

2. Tear basil leaves and add to tomato mixture.

{ VARIATION:
Add chunks of fresh mozzarella or 1 small sautéed zucchini. }

Exchanges/Choices		
1 Vegetable	Calories 30	Potassium 260 mg
	Calories from Fat 15 g	Total Carbohydrate 5 g
	Total Fat 1.5 g	Dietary Fiber 1 g
	Saturated Fat 0.2 g	Sugars 3 g
	Trans Fat 0.0 g	Protein 1 g
	Cholesterol 0 mg	Phosphorus 30 mg
	Sodium 155 mg	

Portobello Mushrooms & Onions with Balsamic Glaze

SERVES: 15 / SERVING SIZE: 1/15 RECIPE

This sautéed mushroom mixture is great as a Bruschetta topping, a side dish for a grilled protein, or a pasta topping. It can even be served as an appetizer or hors d'oeuvre. This great recipe can be made a day ahead of time and reheated or brought to room temperature before serving.

» 2 teaspoons olive oil
» 2 cups onion, thinly sliced
» 2 garlic cloves, minced
» 6 Portobello mushrooms, sliced 1/4-inch thick, or 16 ounces of any mushroom
» Sea salt to taste
» Freshly ground pepper to taste
» Crushed red pepper to taste (optional)
» 3/4 cup balsamic vinegar

1. Heat a sauté pan and thinly film with olive oil. Add onion, garlic, and mushrooms. Cook until soft and onions are translucent. Add salt and pepper to taste and red pepper, if desired.

2. Heat balsamic vinegar in a small saucepan, bring to a boil, and reduce to low. Cook until syrupy, or the vinegar lightly coats the back of a spoon, about 20 minutes. Set aside.

3. Spread mushroom mixture on grilled bread and drizzle with balsamic vinegar.

Exchanges/Choices
1 Vegetable

Calories 30
   Calories from Fat 5
Total Fat 0.5 g
   Saturated Fat 0.1 g
   Trans Fat 0.0 g
Cholesterol 0 mg
Sodium 5 mg

Potassium 170 mg
Total Carbohydrate 5 g
   Dietary Fiber 0 g
   Sugars 3 g
Protein 1 g
Phosphorus 40 mg

Roasted Garlic

SERVES: 6 / SERVING SIZE: 1 TABLESPOON

Roasted garlic is great to have on-hand to add rich flavor to sauces and dressings. It is also great as a Bruschetta topping.

» 4 large heads of garlic
» 1 teaspoon extra virgin olive oil
» 1/2 teaspoon fine sea salt
» Freshly ground pepper

{ VARIATION: Break cloves apart, drizzle with oil, season with salt and pepper, and roast in foil 20–30 minutes. }

1. Preheat oven to 400°F.

2. Using chef's knife, slice a thin piece off the top or stem end of the garlic to expose most of the cloves.

3. Place garlic on large sheet of aluminum foil and drizzle with just enough olive oil to moisten the garlic, approximately 1/4 teaspoon per head.

4. Sprinkle with a dash of sea salt and freshly ground pepper.

5. Wrap up tightly and place in ceramic dish. Bake approximately 45 minutes or until very soft to the touch and a spreadable consistency. Let cool. Squeeze from skins and mash to a puréed consistency. Refrigerate and use as needed.

Exchanges/Choices	Calories 60	Potassium 145 mg
1 Carbohydrate	Calories from Fat 10	Total Carbohydrate 12 g
	Total Fat 1.0 g	Dietary Fiber 1 g
	Saturated Fat 0.1 g	Sugars 0 g
	Trans Fat 0.0 g	Protein 2 g
	Cholesterol 0 mg	Phosphorus 55 mg
	Sodium 205 mg	

White Bean, Herbs, Garlic, and Lemon Spread

SERVES: 10 / SERVING SIZE: 1/4 CUP

This dip is similar to hummus; however, I left out the Tahini (sesame paste), which is almost all fat and can be costly and not readily available. It also has a brighter, fresher flavor. Serve it as a dip for pita chips and raw vegetables or as a spread for Bruschetta or grilled vegetable sandwiches. This dish can be prepared up to two days ahead of time.

» 2 cups canned chickpeas or white beans, drained and rinsed well
» 2 cloves garlic, crushed and peeled
» 2 lemons, juiced
» 1 tablespoon extra virgin olive oil
» 1/2 teaspoon fine sea salt
» 1/4 teaspoon freshly ground pepper
» 1/4 cup chopped Italian parsley
» 1 tablespoon chopped fresh chives

1. Mix all ingredients, except parsley and chives, in a food processor to make a smooth paste. Remove from food processor and stir in fresh herbs.

{ COOK'S TIP:
To crush and peel garlic at the same time, you can place it on a cutting board and crush it with the side of a large chef's knife of a flat meat pounder. }

Exchanges/Choices		
1/2 Starch	Calories 65	Potassium 105 mg
1/2 Fat	Calories from Fat 20	Total Carbohydrate 9 g
	Total Fat 2.0 g	Dietary Fiber 2 g
	Saturated Fat 0.3 g	Sugars 2 g
	Trans Fat 0.0 g	Protein 3 g
	Cholesterol 0 mg	Phosphorus 55 mg
	Sodium 175 mg	

Chicken Lettuce Wraps

SERVES: 6 / SERVING SIZE: 1 WRAP

Quick and simple—but they don't taste it or look it! This is also a great way to use leftover grilled or roasted chicken. You can even let your guests assemble their own lettuce wraps.

» 6 large lettuce leaves, Boston or Bib lettuce work well
» 6 ounces grilled chicken, finely chopped—see recipe for Basic Grilled Chicken, page 157
» 6 teaspoons Asian peanut sauce
» 6 teaspoons julienne or matchstick carrots
» 2 scallions, thinly sliced

1. Place all ingredients in separate bowls.

2. Begin by laying a piece of lettuce on a plate. Top with chicken, peanut sauce, carrots, and scallions. Roll to enclose filling.

Exchanges/Choices		
1 Lean Meat	Calories 65	Potassium 125 mg
1/2 Fat	Calories from Fat 20	Total Carbohydrate 2 g
	Total Fat 2.5 g	Dietary Fiber 0 g
	Saturated Fat 0.6 g	Sugars 1 g
	Trans Fat 0.0 g	Protein 9 g
	Cholesterol 25 mg	Phosphorus 65 mg
	Sodium 95 mg	

Basil Spinach Cream

SERVES: 6 / SERVING SIZE: 1/6 RECIPE

This recipe makes a very flavorful and really healthy low-fat dip or spread. Your guests won't believe how good it is for them! Serve with fresh veggies, whole-grain crackers, or use as a light sauce on your favorite grilled protein.

» 1 cup fresh baby spinach
» 2 cloves garlic, minced
» 1 tablespoon minced shallot, approximately 1 large
» 1/4 cup grated Parmigiano-Reggiano
» 1/2 cup fresh basil
» 1 cup nonfat cottage cheese
» 2 teaspoons extra virgin olive oil
» 2 tablespoons skim milk (optional)

1. Place spinach, garlic, shallot, Parmigiano-Reggiano and basil in food processor. Process until mixture becomes a fine paste.

2. With motor running, add cottage cheese and oil. Process until smooth. Add milk to achieve the desired consistency.

{ **COOK'S TIP:**
This is even more flavorful when made a day ahead of time. }

Exchanges/Choices
1 Lean Meat

Calories 60
   Calories from Fat 20
Total Fat 2.5 g
   Saturated Fat 0.9 g
   Trans Fat 0.0 g
Cholesterol 5 mg
Sodium 150 mg

Potassium 135 mg
Total Carbohydrate 4 g
   Dietary Fiber 0 g
   Sugars 1 g
Protein 5 g
Phosphorus 100 mg

Devilled Eggs

SERVES: 12 / SERVING SIZE: 1/2 LARGE EGG

Devilled eggs are a classic treat! With creative garnishes like sliced grape tomatoes, olives, radish slices, scallions, caviar, or truffle paste, they can be varied in many creative ways.

» 6 large eggs
» 2 tablespoons, plus 1 teaspoon light mayonnaise
» 1/8 teaspoon dry mustard
» Pinch of salt
» Freshly ground black pepper

1. Place the eggs in a small saucepan so that they won't bounce or move around and crack. Cover with water. Bring to a boil. Immediately turn off and cover. Let sit 15–18 minutes to continue cooking. Pour out the hot water. Shake the eggs in the pan to crack the shells. Add cold water and let sit. (This will make them easier to peel.)

2. Peel the eggs and cut them in half vertically. Remove yolks, place them in a small bowl, and mash with a fork. Add mayo, mustard, salt, and pepper. Fill egg whites with mixture. Garnish with sliced grape tomatoes, sliced olives, sliced radishes, sliced scallions, or a drop of caviar or truffle paste (optional).

Exchanges/Choices		
1 Fat	Calories 45	Potassium 35 mg
	Calories from Fat 25	Total Carbohydrate 1 g
	Total Fat 3.0 g	Dietary Fiber 0 g
	Saturated Fat 0.9 g	Sugars 0 g
	Trans Fat 0.0 g	Protein 3 g
	Cholesterol 95 mg	Phosphorus 50 mg
	Sodium 70 mg	

Stuffed Artichokes

SERVES: 12/ SERVING SIZE: 1/2 ARTICHOKE

I am often asked how to make stuffed artichokes and most people are surprised at how easy it is!

» 6 medium or four large fresh artichokes
» Large bowl of water
» 2 lemons

Stuffing
» 1/4 pound pancetta, finely diced (bacon or any ham of your choice can also be used)
» 1 clove garlic, finely minced
» 1/4 cup toasted Pignoli nuts (pine nuts), chopped
» 1 cup fresh bread crumbs
» 1/4 cup minced fresh parley
» 1/8 teaspoon fine sea salt
» Few grinds freshly ground black pepper
» 3 tablespoons freshly grated Parmigiano-Reggiano
» 1/2 tablespoon extra virgin olive oil

1. Prepare acidulated water. Squeeze lemons into a large bowl of water. (This keeps artichokes from turning brown).

2. Cut stems from artichokes, peel off any tough outer leaves, and trim remaining leaves. Place each artichoke in acidulated water while cleaning remaining artichokes.

3. Place artichokes right side up and fill pan halfway with water. Cook approximately 40 minutes until artichokes are tender and leaves can be easily removed.

4. While artichokes are cooling, preheat the oven to 400°F.

(Continued on next page)

Exchanges/Choices
1/2 Carbohydrate
1 Fat

Calories 105	Potassium 250 mg
Calories from Fat 55	Total Carbohydrate 10 g
Total Fat 6.0 g	Dietary Fiber 5 g
Saturated Fat 1.5 g	Sugars 1 g
Trans Fat 0.0 g	Protein 5 g
Cholesterol 10 mg	Phosphorus 120 mg
Sodium 265 mg	

(Stuffed Artichokes Contined)

5. Remove from pan, drain, and cool until you can handle. Gently open artichoke and remove choke (fuzzy bottom). A grapefruit spoon works well.

6. Place pancetta in large sauté pan. Cook until crisp. Add garlic and nuts. Cook until garlic is fragrant. Add bread crumbs, parsley, salt, and pepper. Cool. Add cheese.

7. Stuff each artichoke and place stuffed artichokes in baking dish.

8. Drizzle with extra virgin olive oil. Bake until golden, approximately 20 minutes.

Spiedini with Speck, Asiago, Figs, Shrimp & Balsamico

SERVES: 6 / SERVING SIZE: 1 SKEWER

This beautiful dish is a show stopper. It uses so many wonderful flavors that complement each other. It is also perfect for entertaining because you can prepare it ahead of time and serve it cold.

» 6 wooden skewers (10 inches long)
» 6 pieces (1 ounce total) Asiago Fresco, about 1-inch square each
» 6 slices of speck, about 1 1/2 ounces
» 24 medium to large shrimp, peeled and deveined
» 6 ripe figs, cut in half
» 2 tablespoons good quality, aged balsamic vinegar

{ **COOK'S TIP:**
This dish can be served hot or cold. If you want to do the grilling ahead of serving time, feel free to serve it cold. }

1. Soak the skewers for at least 20 minutes. (This will prevent charring when grilling.)

2. Preheat a grill or grill pan.

3. Wrap each piece of the Asiago in a piece of Speck. Begin making the skewers by threading: two shrimp that have been intertwined to look like one, one fig half, one Speck-wrapped piece of Asiago Fresco, two shrimp that have been intertwined to look like one, and one fig half. Grill until shrimp are pink on one side. Turn and grill until pink on the second side.

4. Place skewers on a platter and drizzle with vinegar. Garnish with additional grated Asiago, if desired.

Exchanges/Choices		
1 Fruit	Calories 100	Potassium 205 mg
1 Lean Meat	Calories from Fat 20	Total Carbohydrate 11 g
	Total Fat 2.5 g	Dietary Fiber 2 g
	Saturated Fat 1.3 g	Sugars 4 g
	Trans Fat 0.0 g	Protein 9 g
	Cholesterol 45 mg	Phosphorus 110 mg
	Sodium 360 mg	

Stuffed Figs

If you prepare this dish when figs are in season, they are both beautiful and delicious. Add them to a salad for an extra special touch. These can be prepared early in the day, covered, and refrigerated.

» 6 ripe figs (soft to the touch)
» 1 1/2 teaspoons spreadable blue cheese
» 12 walnut halves

1. Wash and dry figs. Remove stems.

2. Cut in half vertically.

3. Top with 1/8 teaspoon blue cheese and a walnut half.

Exchanges/Choices		
1/2 Fruit	Calories 35	Potassium 70 mg
	Calories from Fat 15	Total Carbohydrate 5 g
	Total Fat 1.5 g	Dietary Fiber 1 g
	Saturated Fat 0.2 g	Sugars 2 g
	Trans Fat 0.0 g	Protein 1 g
	Cholesterol 0 mg	Phosphorus 10 mg
	Sodium 0 mg	

Mushroom Filled Phyllo Triangles

SERVES: 12 / SERVING SIZE: 1 TRIANGLE

My daughter-in-law and I developed this recipe together for a family gathering and it was a huge hit!

» 5 (14 × 18-inch) sheets phyllo
» 10 ounces cremini mushrooms
» 1 large shallot
» 2 small garlic cloves
» 1/2 teaspoon fine sea salt
» Few grinds black pepper
» 1/4 cup herbs (such as thyme and basil)
» Nonstick cooking spray or olive oil mister
» 3 ounces light herb cheese spread, such as Rondele or Boursin

1. Defrost Phyllo in refrigerator at least 3 hours. (Do not defrost in microwave as it will become gummy.)

2. Wipe mushrooms with damp paper towel to remove any debris. Cut a fine sliver off the end of the stem and quarter the mushrooms. Peel and quarter the shallot. Crush and peel garlic.

3. Fit food processor with steel blade. Place mushrooms, shallots, and garlic in food processor. Pulse to a finely chopped mixture. Add salt, pepper, and herbs and pulse again.

4. Thinly film a sauté pan with extra virgin olive oil and cook mushroom mixture until soft, approximately 5 minutes. Turn off heat, add cheese spread, and mix well.

(Continued on next page)

Exchanges/Choices
1/2 Starch

Calories 55
   Calories from Fat 15
Total Fat 1.5 g
   Saturated Fat 0.4 g
   Trans Fat 0.0 g
Cholesterol 0 mg
Sodium 170 mg

Potassium 150 mg
Total Carbohydrate 8 g
   Dietary Fiber 1 g
   Sugars 1 g
Protein 2 g
Phosphorus 50 mg

(Mushroom Filled Phyllo Triangles Continued)

5. Unwrap defrosted phyllo and lay it on parchment-lined work surface. Cover with plastic wrap and a damp towel to prevent it from drying out.

6. Spray phyllo with cooking spray or olive oil and add another piece of phyllo. Repeat with remaining phyllo. Cut into 2-inch strips. Place one teaspoon of mushroom mixture on the bottom end of Phyllo and fold a triangle shape over the rest of the Phyllo. Repeat until you have wrapped the length of Phyllo and made a triangle. (Think of it like folding a flag.)

7. Place triangles on a parchment-lined baking sheet. Baked at 375°F for 8–10 minutes.

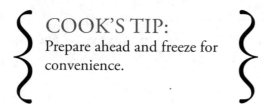

COOK'S TIP:
Prepare ahead and freeze for convenience.

Grilled Vegetable Quesadilla with Roasted Corn Salsa

SERVES: 8 / SERVING SIZE: 1 QUESADILLA

This recipe is a great way to use leftover grilled veggies for a light meal or a quick snack.

Roasted Corn Salsa

» 1 ear fresh (uncooked) corn, kernels cut from cob
» 1 red bell pepper, chopped
» 1 cup sliced cherry or grape tomatoes
» 1/2 cup cilantro, roughly chopped
» 1 clove garlic, crushed and minced
» 1 lime, juiced

» Grilled Vegetables (page 103)
» 8 large whole-wheat tortillas
» 2 cups shredded Cabot 75% reduced-fat cheddar cheese

1. Preheat oven to 375°F.

2. Heat a large dry sauté pan over medium heat. Add corn and roast over high heat, shaking pan. When corn begins to brown, add pepper, tomatoes, cilantro, garlic, and lime juice and cook on low heat for 5 minutes.

3. Roughly chop Grilled Vegetables.

4. Cover half of each tortilla with chopped, Grilled Vegetables and top with 1/4 cup cheese. Fold tortillas and place on baking sheet. Bake until golden brown, about 10 minutes. Cut into wedges and top with Roasted Corn Salsa.

Exchanges/Choices
2 Starch
4 Vegetable
1 Med-Fat Meat

Calories 325
  Calories from Fat 65
Total Fat 7.0 g
  Saturated Fat 2.2 g
  Trans Fat 0.0 g
Cholesterol 10 mg
Sodium 615 mg

Potassium 730 mg
Total Carbohydrate 53 g
  Dietary Fiber 9 g
  Sugars 11 g
Protein 17 g
Phosphorus 330 mg

Oven-Baked Herb Onion Rings

SERVES: 4 / SERVING SIZE: 1/4 RECIPE

» 1 teaspoon extra virgin olive oil
» 1/4 cup panko
» 2 tablespoons Parmigiano-Reggiano
» 1 teaspoon signature herb blend or Italian herb blend (See Tips, page 7)
» 2 large onions, sliced into 1/4–1/2-inch rounds

1. Preheat oven to 400°F.

2. Mix olive oil, panko, Parmigiano, and herb blend in large bowl. Add onions and toss to mix well.

3. Place on parchment-lined baking sheet and bake until edges are browned, approximately 15 minutes.

Exchanges/Choices
2 Vegetable
1/2 Fat

Calories 80
   Calories from Fat 20
Total Fat 2.0 g
   Saturated Fat 0.7 g
   Trans Fat 0.0 g
Cholesterol 0 mg
Sodium 25 mg

Potassium 175 mg
Total Carbohydrate 14 g
   Dietary Fiber 2 g
   Sugars 5 g
Protein 2 g
Phosphorus 55 mg

Turkey Kebabs with Avocado & Tomato

SERVES: 9 / SERVING SIZE: 2 KABOBS

Serve these colorful Turkey Kebabs with the Mango Dipping Sauce on page 29 (optional).

» Juice of 1 lime, plus additional juice for finishing
» 1/2 teaspoon fine sea salt
» 1/4 teaspoon freshly ground black pepper
» 1 teaspoon extra virgin olive oil
» 2 garlic cloves, minced
» 3/4 pound turkey tenderloin or turkey medallions, cut into 36, 1-inch cubes
» 9 cherry tomatoes
» 1 ripe avocado

1. Mix together the lime juice, salt, pepper, olive oil, and garlic. Place this mixture and the turkey in a plastic bag and marinate in the fridge for at least 20 minutes.

2. Cut tomatoes in half vertically. Cut the avocado into 18 chunks.

3. Grill or broil the turkey. Set aside to cool.

4. Thread the kebabs as follows: 1 piece of turkey, 1 piece of tomato, 1 piece of turkey, and 1 piece of avocado

5. Squeeze lime over kebabs and serve with a drizzle of Mango Dipping Sauce, page 29 (optional).

Exchanges/Choices		
1 Lean Meat	Calories 75	Potassium 210 mg
1/2 Fat	Calories from Fat 25	Total Carbohydrate 3 g
	Total Fat 3.0 g	Dietary Fiber 1 g
	Saturated Fat 0.5 g	Sugars 1 g
	Trans Fat 0.0 g	Protein 9 g
	Cholesterol 25 mg	Phosphorus 80 mg
	Sodium 150 mg	

Mango Dipping Sauce

SERVES: 10 / SERVING SIZE: 1/10 RECIPE

This versatile dipping sauce is very flavorful and can be served with several dishes in this book, baked chips, or any simple grilled protein.

» 1 ripe mango
» 6 ounces low-fat Greek yogurt, pineapple variety
» Juice of 1 lime
» 1/2 teaspoon honey
» 1/4 teaspoon togarashi seasoning (Japanese dry spice powder)
» 1/2 cup chopped fresh cilantro

1. Cut mango into large chunks. Place in food processor and chop. Add yogurt, lime juice, honey, togarashi, and cilantro. Process to a paste. Refrigerate and let flavors blend for at least 30 minutes.

2. Serve as a dipping sauce with chips, vegetables, or Turkey Kebabs with Avocado and Tomato, page 28.

Exchanges/Choices		
1/2 Carbohydrate	Calories 35	Potassium 80 mg
	Calories from Fat 0	Total Carbohydrate 7 g
	Total Fat 0.0 g	Dietary Fiber 0 g
	Saturated Fat 0.2 g	Sugars 6 g
	Trans Fat 0.0 g	Protein 1 g
	Cholesterol 0 mg	Phosphorus 25 mg
	Sodium 10 mg	

CHAPTER 3:
Salads

The Stress Free Diabetes Kitchen

Salads

Orzo, Lentil, and Fig Salad

SERVES: 8 / SERVING SIZE: 1/8 RECIPE

The delicious and healthy flavors of the Mediterranean inspired me to create this salad. This recipe can be made a day or two ahead of time and kept refrigerated. This recipe is great for picnics, make-ahead meals, or brown bag lunches.

» 8 ounces uncooked Orzo (rice shaped pasta), or the pasta shape of your choice
» 1 cup uncooked lentils, preferably French or small dark green
» 1/2 cup oil-cured black olives, pitted and chopped
» 1/2 cup dried mission figlets, sliced
» 1/2 cup crumbled, fat-free feta cheese
» 1/2 cup toasted pignoli nuts (pine nuts)
» 3 tablespoons white balsamic vinegar
» 6 tablespoons extra virgin olive oil
» 2 cloves garlic, minced
» 1 tablespoon fresh oregano, chopped
» 1/2 cup fresh basil leaves, torn
» Fine sea salt
» Freshly ground black pepper
» Additional herbs for garnish (basil)

1. Cook orzo according to package directions, approximately 9 minutes.

2. Cook lentils in 3 cups water until tender, approximately 20 minutes.

3. Place balsamic vinegar in bowl. Add garlic, oregano, basil, a pinch of sea salt, and a few grindings of pepper. Slowly whisk in olive oil. Set aside.

4. Mix orzo, lentils, olives, figs, cheese, and nuts together. Add dressing. Taste and adjust seasonings.

5. Garnish with fresh herbs before serving.

Exchanges/Choices		
2 Starch	Calories 395	Potassium 415 mg
1 Fruit	Calories from Fat 180	Total Carbohydrate 44 g
1 Lean Meat	Total Fat 20.0 g	Dietary Fiber 8 g
3 Fat	Saturated Fat 2.2 g	Sugars 10 g
	Trans Fat 0.0 g	Protein 13 g
	Cholesterol 0 mg	Phosphorus 250 mg
	Sodium 435 mg	

Frisee, Fennel and Orange Salad

SERVES: 8 / SERVING SIZE: 1/8 RECIPE

This salad is so beautiful and tasty you will want it with every meal. It's also great with leftover sliced meats like the Roasted Filet Mignon (page 173) or Roast Chicken with Preserved Lemons (page 160). You can also use a variety of greens, nuts, and cheese that compliment the rest of the meal.

» 1/4 cup pignoli nuts (pine nuts), toasted
» 1 large bulb fennel, sliced thinly
» 2 cups baby spinach
» 1 medium head Frisée or green leaf lettuce
» 2 tablespoons crumbled gorgonzola cheese
» 2 tablespoons balsamic vinegar
» 1/4 cup extra virgin olive oil
» 1 drop orange oil or orange extract
» 1 10-ounce can mandarin oranges, drained

1. Toast nuts by placing them in a small, dry skillet and cooking until golden. Remove from pan and cool.

2. Wash and dry fennel, spinach, and lettuce and place in a large salad bowl. Top with crumbled gorgonzola cheese and toasted pignoli nuts.

3. Place vinegar in medium-size bowl. Slowly whisk in olive oil until mixture has been emulsified to a creamy texture. Add orange oil.

4. Add dressing to greens in small amounts and toss well. Add oranges and toss gently.

{ COOK'S TIP:
Salad should not be swimming in dressing. It's better to add less and decide you need more. }

Exchanges/Choices		
1/2 Carbohydrate	Calories 125	Potassium 330 mg
2 Fat	Calories from Fat 90	Total Carbohydrate 7 g
	Total Fat 10.0 g	Dietary Fiber 2 g
	Saturated Fat 1.5 g	Sugars 3 g
	Trans Fat 0.0 g	Protein 2 g
	Cholesterol 0 mg	Phosphorus 65 mg
	Sodium 70 mg	

Fresh Tomato and Basil Salad

SERVES: 4 / SERVING SIZE: 1/4 RECIPE

Make this salad a few hours ahead so the flavors really have a chance to meld. You can also use this as a Bruschetta topping—just cut the tomatoes into very small pieces.

» Plum tomatoes, roughly chopped, or 2 cups cherry tomatoes, halved
» 2 cloves garlic, chopped
» 1 shallot, minced, or 1 small red onion, chopped
» 2 tablespoons extra virgin olive oil
» 1/2 teaspoon fine sea salt
» Freshly ground pepper
» 1 tablespoon red wine vinegar (optional)
» 1 cup fresh basil leaves

1. Mix tomatoes, garlic, and shallot. Add olive oil, salt, and pepper. Taste for seasoning and add vinegar, if desired.

2. Tear basil leaves and add to tomato mixture. Serve at room temperature.

VARIATION:
For bruschetta: slice a loaf of good Italian bread. Grill or broil until browned and then brush with extra virgin olive oil and rub with a cut clove of garlic.

Exchanges/Choices		
2 Vegetable	Calories 105	Potassium 555 mg
1 1/2 Fat	Calories from Fat 65	Total Carbohydrate 10 g
	Total Fat 7.0 g	Dietary Fiber 3 g
	Saturated Fat 1.0 g	Sugars 6 g
	Trans Fat 0.0 g	Protein 2 g
	Cholesterol 0 mg	Phosphorus 60 mg
	Sodium 305 mg	

Tre Colore Salad with Basic Vinaigrette

SERVES: 6 / SERVING SIZE: 1/6 RECIPE

This salad is perfect as a side dish or topped with grilled chicken for a full meal. Use a variety of greens—spring mix or baby spinach—or add cheeses and nuts that complement the rest of the meal.

» 1 head green leaf lettuce
» 1 small head radicchio
» 1 medium head Belgian endive
» Half a pomegranate, seeds only
» 1 recipe Basic Vinaigrette (see page 37)

1. Wash and dry salad ingredients. Tear and place in large salad bowl. Add Vinaigrette in small amounts and toss well.

COOK'S TIP:
Salad should not be swimming in dressing. It's better to add less and decide you need more. Drying the greens in a salad spinner helps the dressing cling to the greens.

Exchanges/Choices		
1 Vegetable	Calories 70	Potassium 260 mg
1 Fat	Calories from Fat 45	Total Carbohydrate 6 g
	Total Fat 5.0 g	Dietary Fiber 2 g
	Saturated Fat 0.7 g	Sugars 3 g
	Trans Fat 0.0 g	Protein 1 g
	Cholesterol 0 mg	Phosphorus 35 mg
	Sodium 30 mg	

Basic Vinaigrette

SERVES: 12 / SERVING SIZE: 1 TABLESPOON

Basic vinaigrette can also be used as a salad dressing or as a marinade.

» 1/4 cup vinegar
» Fresh herbs such as chives or basil, chopped
» Pinch fine sea salt
» Freshly ground pepper, to taste
» 1/2 cup extra virgin olive oil

1. Place vinegar, herbs, salt, and pepper in bowl. Start whisking and slowly stream in the olive oil. Taste after 1/2 cup has been added. (The amount of oil required to balance the vinegar will depend on the vinegar selected.)

VARIATION:
» Use different types and flavors of vinegar.
» Add 1–2 drops orange oil or orange extract.
» Add chopped fresh herbs or roasted garlic.
» Add fresh raspberries or crushed cranberries.

Exchanges/Choices		
2 Fat	Calories 80	Potassium 0 mg
	Calories from Fat 80	Total Carbohydrate 0 g
	Total Fat 9.0 g	Dietary Fiber 0 g
	Saturated Fat 1.2 g	Sugars 0 g
	Trans Fat 0.0 g	Protein 0 g
	Cholesterol 0 mg	Phosphorus 0 mg
	Sodium 10 mg	

Orzo Salad with Roasted Eggplant, Zucchini & Red Pepper

SERVES: 12 / SERVING SIZE: 1/12 RECIPE

Orzo is rice-shaped pasta that holds up well in salads and is bite-sized, which works well for parties.

» 16 ounces uncooked orzo or the pasta shape of your choice
» 1 cup uncooked lentils, preferably French or small dark green
» 4 cups Roasted Vegetables (page 104)
» 2 cloves garlic, minced, divided use
» 1/2 cup extra virgin olive oil, divided use
» Fine sea salt
» Freshly ground black pepper
» 1/4 cup white balsamic vinegar
» 1 tablespoon fresh oregano, chopped
» 1/2 cup fresh basil leaves, torn
» 1/2 cup oil cured black olives, pitted and chopped
» 1 cup crumbled fat-free feta cheese
» 1/2 cup toasted Pignoli nuts (pine nuts)
» Additional herbs for garnish (basil)

1. Cook orzo according to package directions, approximately 9 minutes.

2. Cook lentils in 3 cups water until tender, approximately 20 minutes.

3. Roast veggies (see page 104).

4. Preheat oven to 425°F.

5. Salt veggies on both sides and let stand for 10–20 minutes. This will prevent them from absorbing too much oil.

6. Line baking sheet with parchment. Place cut vegetables and garlic in large bowl. Drizzle with small amount of olive oil. Toss. Place on baking sheet. Sprinkle with salt and pepper to taste.

(Continued on next page)

Exchanges/Choices		
2 1/2 Starch	Calories 370	Potassium 375 mg
1 Vegetable	Calories from Fat 155	Total Carbohydrate 44 g
1 Lean Meat	Total Fat 17.0 g	Dietary Fiber 7 g
2 1/2 Fat	Saturated Fat 2.0 g	Sugars 8 g
	Trans Fat 0.0 g	Protein 13 g
	Cholesterol 0 mg	Phosphorus 225 mg
	Sodium 475 mg	

(Orzo Salad with Roasted Eggplant, Zucchini, & Red Pepper Continued)

7. Roast to desired doneness, approximately 20–30 minutes. Set aside.

8. Place balsamic in bowl. Add garlic, oregano, basil, a pinch of sea salt, and a few grindings of pepper. Slowly whisk in olive oil. Set aside.

9. Mix orzo, lentils, olives, roasted veggies, cheese, and nuts together. Add dressing. Taste and adjust seasonings. Garnish with fresh herbs before serving.

COOK'S TIP:
Great for picnics, make-ahead meals, or brown bag lunches. It can even be made a day or two ahead and kept refrigerated.

Green Market Salad with Raspberries & Edible Flowers

SERVES: 6 / SERVING SIZE: 1/6 RECIPE

A simple trip to the Farmer's Market is all you need to gather all the ingredients for this beautiful salad. Use a variety of greens, spring mix, or baby spinach. Add cheeses and nuts to complement the meal.

» 1 head green leaf lettuce
» 1 small head radicchio
» 1 medium head Belgian endive
» 1 recipe Basic Vinaigrette (page 37)
» 1 cup fresh raspberries
» Edible flowers

1. Wash and dry first three ingredients. Tear lettuce, radicchio, and endive and place in large salad bowl.

2. Add dressing in small amounts and toss well. Top with raspberries and flowers.

COOK'S TIP:
» Drying the greens in a salad spinner will help the dressing cling to the greens.
» Flowers should be placed on top because they are so delicate.

Exchanges/Choices		
1 Vegetable	Calories 65	Potassium 260 mg
1 Fat	Calories from Fat 45	Total Carbohydrate 6 g
	Total Fat 5.0 g	Dietary Fiber 3 g
	Saturated Fat 0.7 g	Sugars 1 g
	Trans Fat 0.0 g	Protein 1 g
	Cholesterol 0 mg	Phosphorus 35 mg
	Sodium 30 mg	

Pasta Salad with Figs & Prosciutto

SERVES: 8 / SERVING SIZE: 1/8 RECIPE

» 1 pound mini bow tie pasta, cooked al dente
» 2 ounces imported prosciutto, cut into bite-size pieces
» 4 ounces dried figs, stems removed and sliced in half
» 3/4 cup shredded Asiago cheese
» 1 clove garlic, minced finely or mashed to a paste
» Pinch of sea salt
» Few grindings black pepper
» 2 tablespoons white balsamic vinegar
» 1/4 cup extra virgin olive oil
» 1/2 cup basil leaves, thinly sliced or chopped
» 24 grape tomatoes

1. Place pasta, prosciutto, figs, and cheese together in a large salad bowl.

2. Whisk together the garlic, salt, pepper, and vinegar. Slowly whisk in the oil until well blended.

3. Pour over the salad bowl and toss well. Add the basil and gently mix in. Top each serving with three tomatoes.

4. Serve chilled or at room temperature.

{ COOK'S TIP:
Al dente means "to the tooth." Your pasta should be firm when you bite into it. }

Exchanges/Choices		
3 Starch	Calories 350	Potassium 250 mg
1/2 Fruit	Calories from Fat 90	Total Carbohydrate 53 g
1 Med-Fat Meat	Total Fat 10.0 g	Dietary Fiber 4 g
1/2 Fat	Saturated Fat 2.5 g	Sugars 11 g
	Trans Fat 0.0 g	Protein 11 g
	Cholesterol 10 mg	Phosphorus 155 mg
	Sodium 200 mg	

Endive, Apple & Walnut Salad with Frico

SERVES 4 / SERVING SIZE: 1/4 RECIPE

A Frico is a crispy cheese round that is a wonderful, tasty treat. This salad is also great with leftover sliced meats, such as Filet Mignon with Shrimp & Red Wine Reduction (page 173) or Enlightened Herb Roast Chicken with Garlic & Lemon (page 160).

Frico
» 1 1/2 cups Grana Padano cheese, coarsely grated
» Freshly ground black pepper

» 4 walnut halves

Salad
» 2 large Belgian endive
» 1 large tart apple
» 1 lemon, juiced
» 1 tablespoon balsamic vinegar
» 1 1/2 tablespoon extra virgin olive oil
» 1 drop orange oil or orange extract
» 4 small whole-wheat rolls

1. Preheat oven 350°F.

2. In a bowl, combine grated cheese with freshly ground black pepper.

3. Line two sheet pans with a Silpat or other nonstick surface.

4. Measure out 1 tablespoon of grated cheese and spread into 1 1/2-inch rounds on prepared sheet pan. Continue making rounds with the cheese mixture until all the cheese is used. Bake for 6–7 minutes or until golden.

5. Toast nuts by placing in a small dry skillet and cooking until golden. Remove from pan and cool. Place in plastic bag and roughly chop.

(Continued on next page)

Exchanges/Choices
1 Starch
1/2 Fruit
1 Vegetable
2 Fat

Calories 215
    Calories from Fat 90
Total Fat 10.0 g
    Saturated Fat 2.5 g
    Trans Fat 0.0 g
Cholesterol 5 mg
Sodium 235 mg

Potassium 385 mg
Total Carbohydrate 28 g
    Dietary Fiber 5 g
    Sugars 9 g
Protein 6 g
Phosphorus 145 mg

6. Wash and dry endive. Thinly slice lengthwise. Wash apple and thinly slice. Sprinkle with lemon juice to prevent browning.

7. Place vinegar in medium-size bowl. Slowly whisk in olive oil until mixture has been emulsified to a creamy texture. Add orange oil.

8. Place endive and apple sliced on individual salad plates or a large platter. Drizzle with dressing. Top with nuts and 1 serving of Frico (remaining Frico can be stored in an airtight container for later use). Serve with whole-wheat rolls.

{ VARIATION:
Use a variety of greens. Select cheeses and nuts that complement the rest of the meal. }

Asparagus & Prosciutto Antipasto Salad

SERVES 6 / SERVING SIZE: 1/6 RECIPE

A composed salad is always elegant and this is one of those show stoppers for your special dinner.

Vinaigrette
- » 1 tablespoon white wine vinegar
- » Pinch fine sea salt
- » 3–4 grindings of freshly milled black pepper
- » 2 tablespoons extra virgin olive oil
- » 1 tablespoon fresh herbs (chives, basil, or parsley)
- » 1 teaspoon orange zest (optional)

- » 3 slices prosciutto (cut in half)
- » 1/2 pound roasted or steamed asparagus
- » 1 orange, sliced
- » 6 dried figs
- » 1/4 cup Italian olive mix
- » 1/2 ounce Parmigiano-Reggiano

1. Place vinegar, salt, and pepper in a small to medium mixing bowl. Slowly whisk in extra virgin olive oil. Whisk until well blended. Stir in herbs and zest, if desired. Set aside to use on the salad.

2. To plate the salad, you will need a large dinner plate. Begin by placing the prosciutto in a single layer on the plate. Top with the asparagus spears; add oranges, figs, and olives. Use a vegetable peeler to "peel" off slices of the cheese and place on top of the salad.

3. Drizzle with vinaigrette and serve with bread or breadsticks.

Exchanges/Choices		
1/2 Fruit	Calories 110	Potassium 180 mg
1 1/2 Fat	Calories from Fat 65	Total Carbohydrate 10 g
	Total Fat 7.0 g	Dietary Fiber 2 g
	Saturated Fat 1.5 g	Sugars 7 g
	Trans Fat 0.0 g	Protein 4 g
	Cholesterol 5 mg	Phosphorus 55 mg
	Sodium 235 mg	

Classic Italian Panzanella Salad (Bread & Tomato Salad)

SERVES: 4 / SERVING SIZE: 1/4 RECIPE

This is a classic Italian salad that I had during my travels throughout Italy. Each cook puts their own touch on the dish, but the main ingredients—tomatoes, bread, celery, and onion—stay the same.

» 2 medium tomatoes, cut into 1-inch cubes, (or 2 cups cherry tomatoes, cut in half)
» 1/2 teaspoon fine sea salt
» 2 cups good quality Italian bread, such as a multigrain Ciabatta
» 1 cup cucumber, quartered lengthwise, and thinly sliced (about 1/2 of an English cucumber)
» 2 stalks celery, sliced 1/2-inch thick
» 1 small red onion, cut in half and thinly sliced
» 1/4 teaspoon freshly ground black pepper
» 2 tablespoons red wine vinegar
» 2 tablespoons extra virgin olive oil
» 1/2 cup fresh basil leaves, torn into strips
» 1 cup flat Italian parsley leaves, roughly chopped

1. Place tomatoes in large salad bowl and sprinkle with salt. Let stand 5 minutes.

2. Break up bread and add to tomatoes. Add remaining salad ingredients and mix well.

Exchanges/Choices		
1 Starch	Calories 160	Potassium 415 mg
1 Vegetable	Calories from Fat 70	Total Carbohydrate 20 g
1 1/2 Fat	Total Fat 8.0 g	Dietary Fiber 3 g
	Saturated Fat 1.2 g	Sugars 4 g
	Trans Fat 0.0 g	Protein 4 g
	Cholesterol 0 mg	Phosphorus 75 mg
	Sodium 455 mg	

Couscous Salad with Roasted Vegetables

SERVES: 8 / SERVING SIZE: 1/8 RECIPE

Large grain couscous gives this dish more texture, but regular couscous with also work. Simply add cooked protein for a complete meal. Frozen shrimp that is cooked and peeled works perfectly for this dish.

- » 2 cups couscous
- » 4 cups low-sodium chicken/vegetable broth
- » 1 small zucchini (2 cups), cut into 1-inch pieces
- » 1 small eggplant (2 cups), chopped into 1-inch pieces
- » 1 large onion, chopped into 1-inch pieces
- » 1 green bell pepper, chopped into 1-inch pieces
- » 8 cloves garlic, peeled but whole
- » 2 tablespoons, plus 1/4 cup extra virgin olive oil
- » 3 plum tomatoes, chopped
- » 1 tablespoon fresh oregano, chopped
- » 1 tablespoon fresh basil, chopped
- » 1/4 cup balsamic vinegar
- » Fresh Italian parsley, chopped

1. Cook couscous according to package directions, using broth instead of water.

2. Place zucchini, eggplant, onion, pepper, and garlic in large bowl. Toss with 2 tablespoons extra virgin olive oil. Place on baking sheet lined with parchment so that they are in one single layer.

3. Roast in 400° oven for 20 minutes or until tender. Cool. Add tomatoes and herbs when vegetables are cooled.

4. Mix couscous and vegetables. Slowly whisk together 1/4 cup oil into vinegar and add to couscous. Mix well. Place on large platter.

5. Garnish with fresh herbs, chopped tomatoes, or sliced oranges.

Exchanges/Choices
2 Starch
1 Vegetable
2 Fat

Calories 275
   Calories from Fat 100
Total Fat 11.0 g
   Saturated Fat 1.6 g
   Trans Fat 0.0 g
Cholesterol 0 mg
Sodium 55 mg

Potassium 395 mg
Total Carbohydrate 38 g
   Dietary Fiber 4 g
   Sugars 4 g
Protein 7 g
Phosphorus 115 mg

Strawberry Orange Salad with Honey Dressing

SERVES: 5 / SERVING SIZE: 1/5 RECIPE

This salad is perfect on a hot day. It will cool you to the core with its crisp, refreshing taste.

Salad

- » 1 pint strawberries
- » 1 large navel orange
- » 1 banana, sliced
- » Juice of 1 lemon
- » Small head green leaf lettuce

Dressing

- » 1 cup low-fat, plain yogurt
- » 1 tablespoon fresh squeezed orange juice
- » 1 tablespoon lemon juice (Meyer lemon, if available)
- » 2 tablespoons honey
- » 1/4 cup minced fresh mint, plus additional
- » 2 sprigs for garnish

1. Slice strawberries. Peel and segment the orange. Slice banana and dip in lemon juice. Mix together in bowl.

2. Wash and spin-dry the lettuce using a salad spinner. Divide lettuce among five plates. Divide fruit between five lettuce-lined plates. For family-style presentation, place lettuce on platter and top with fruit.

3. Mix together dressing ingredients and spoon over fruit.

Exchanges/Choices		
1 1/2 Fruit	Calories 125	Potassium 455 mg
1/2 Carbohydrate	Calories from Fat 10	Total Carbohydrate 27 g
	Total Fat 1.0 g	Dietary Fiber 3 g
	Saturated Fat 0.5 g	Sugars 20 g
	Trans Fat 0.0 g	Protein 4 g
	Cholesterol 5 mg	Phosphorus 115 mg
	Sodium 45 mg	

White Bean Salad with Lemon & Basil

SERVES: 6 / SERVING SIZE: 1/6 RECIPE

These are flavors that were born to be together. You can serve this dish with grilled chicken or fish over mixed greens for a complete meal. This salad can even be made a day or two ahead of time.

» 1/4 cup extra virgin olive oil
» 8 large cloves garlic, sliced lengthwise
» 1 lemon, juiced
» 8 sprigs fresh basil or thyme
» 15 ounces canned small white beans, drained and rinsed well
» 1/2 teaspoon fine sea salt
» 1/4 teaspoon freshly ground pepper
» Lemon slices (for garnish)

1. Heat olive oil in small saucepan. Add sliced garlic and cook until golden. Remove garlic from oil with slotted spoon.

2. Mix olive oil with lemon juice, basil or thyme, and beans. Add salt and pepper to taste. Set aside to allow flavors to blend. Garnish with lemon slices before serving.

Exchanges/Choices		
1 Starch	Calories 145	Potassium 195 mg
1 1/2 Fat	Calories from Fat 80	Total Carbohydrate 13 g
	Total Fat 9.0 g	Dietary Fiber 4 g
	Saturated Fat 1.3 g	Sugars 0 g
	Trans Fat 0.0 g	Protein 4 g
	Cholesterol 0 mg	Phosphorus 65 mg
	Sodium 285 mg	

White Bean & Broccoli Salad with Tomato

SERVES: 6 / SERVING SIZE: 1/6 RECIPE

» 1/4 cup extra virgin olive oil

» 1 head broccoli rabe or broccoli, cut into
2–3-inch pieces or florets

» 1/2 cup low-sodium vegetable stock

» 2 cloves garlic, minced

» 2 cups small white beans, drained and
rinsed

» 6 plum tomatoes, chopped

» 1/2 teaspoon fine sea salt

» 1/4 teaspoon freshly ground pepper

1. Thinly film the sauté pan with olive oil. Add broccoli and stock. Cover and cook 5 minutes. Add minced garlic and white beans and cook 5 minutes. Remove from heat. Add tomatoes. Season with salt and pepper to taste.

2. Sprinkle with balsamic vinegar, if desired. Garnish with grated Parmigiano-Reggiano or Grana Padano, if desired.

{ COOK'S TIP:
Can be served over linguine or with a great loaf of bread. }

Exchanges/Choices		
1 Starch	Calories 195	Potassium 510 mg
1 Vegetable	Calories from Fat 90	Total Carbohydrate 21 g
2 Fat	Total Fat 10.0 g	Dietary Fiber 9 g
	Saturated Fat 1.4 g	Sugars 2 g
	Trans Fat 0.0 g	Protein 7 g
	Cholesterol 0 mg	Phosphorus 150 mg
	Sodium 360 mg	

Cherry Tomato, Scallion & Parsley Salad

SERVES: 4 / SERVING SIZE: 1/4 RECIPE

» 1 pint cherry tomatoes, cut in half
» 1/2 teaspoon fine Italian sea salt with herbs (or plain sea salt)
» 4–6 thin scallions, sliced 1/2-inch thick on the diagonal
» 1 tablespoon extra virgin olive oil
» 2 teaspoons red wine vinegar
» 1/2 cup large Italian parsley leaves
» 1/2 teaspoon black pepper

1. Place tomatoes in large bowl and sprinkle with salt. Let stand for 20 minutes.

2. Add scallions. Drizzle with extra virgin olive oil and red wine vinegar. Toss. Let stand until serving time.

3. Add parsley. Season with black pepper and serve.

{ COOK'S TIP:
Vary this salad by using different herbs, such as basil or cilantro. }

Exchanges/Choices		
1 Vegetable	Calories 50	Potassium 240 mg
1/2 Fat	Calories from Fat 30	Total Carbohydrate 4 g
	Total Fat 3.5 g	Dietary Fiber 1 g
	Saturated Fat 0.5 g	Sugars 2 g
	Trans Fat 0.0 g	Protein 1 g
	Cholesterol 0 mg	Phosphorus 25 mg
	Sodium 305 mg	

Chinese Chicken Salad

SERVES: 6 / SERVING SIZE: 1/6 RECIPE

Chicken
- » 4 pieces boneless, skinless chicken breasts
- » Sea salt, fine grind
- » Freshly ground black pepper

Salad
- » 1 medium head Napa cabbage, julienne, reserve a couple of large leaves for serving
- » 1 small heart of Romaine, julienne
- » Handful of snow peas, julienne
- » 1/2 cup toasted pignoli nuts (pine nuts)

Dressing
- » 2 teaspoons dry mustard
- » 1/4 cup rice wine vinegar
- » 1 teaspoon peanut butter
- » 1 teaspoon soy sauce
- » 1 tablespoon sesame oil
- » 1 tablespoon canola oil
- » Salt to taste
- » Few grinds black pepper

1. Pound chicken breast to even thickness. Season chicken with a pinch of sea salt and pepper. Grill 3-4 minutes on each side. Cool and slice into thin strips.

2. Mix all salad ingredients together in a bowl.

3. Whisk dressing ingredients together. Toss salad greens and dressing together. Add chicken. Serve on large Napa cabbage leaves.

Exchanges/Choices		
1 Vegetable	Calories 240	Potassium 560 mg
3 Lean Meat	Calories from Fat 135	Total Carbohydrate 7 g
2 Fat	Total Fat 15.0 g	Dietary Fiber 3 g
	Saturated Fat 1.7 g	Sugars 3 g
	Trans Fat 0.0 g	Protein 20 g
	Cholesterol 45 mg	Phosphorus 235 mg
	Sodium 300 mg	

Wild Rice & Chicken Salad

SERVES: 8 / SERVING SIZE: 1/8 RECIPE

This is a great summer salad.

» 2 cups wild rice, cooked
» 1 cup seedless red and green grapes
» 1/2 cup Champagne vinegar
» 1/4 cup chopped fresh thyme, plus additional for garnish
» 1/2 cup extra virgin olive oil
» Fine sea salt
» Freshly ground pepper to taste
» 1 pound boneless, skinless chicken or turkey breast, poached, cooled, and diced
» 6 cups baby greens

1. Cook wild rice according to package; this will take approximately 45–60 minutes.

2. If grapes are large they can be sliced in half.

3. Mix Champagne vinegar and thyme. Slowly whisk in olive oil. Season with salt and pepper. Add more oil if dressing tastes too acidic.

4. Combine chicken, rice, and grapes. Season to taste with salt and pepper. Add dressing to taste. Serve over baby greens. Garnish with additional thyme.

Exchanges/Choices		
1 1/2 Starch	Calories 315	Potassium 305 mg
1/2 Carbohydrate	Calories from Fat 135	Total Carbohydrate 28 g
2 Lean Meat	Total Fat 15.0 g	Dietary Fiber 3 g
2 Fat	Saturated Fat 2.3 g	Sugars 4 g
	Trans Fat 0.0 g	Protein 17 g
	Cholesterol 35 mg	Phosphorus 185 mg
	Sodium 60 mg	

Festive Pasta Salad with a Rainbow of Vegetables

SERVES: 8 / SERVING SIZE: 1/8 RECIPE

This is a great dish for kids—they can eat a rainbow! To make it more fun for young kids, use wagon wheel pasta.

1 pound short pasta of your choice
1/2 cup extra virgin olive oil
1/2 cup red wine vinegar
1 clove garlic, minced
1/2 teaspoon fine sea salt
Freshly ground black pepper
1 15-ounce can dark red kidney beans, drained and rinsed
2 cups baby spinach, roughly chopped
1/2 cup black olives, sliced
1 yellow bell pepper, diced
1 red bell pepper, diced

1. Cook pasta according to package directions.

2. Whisk oil and vinegar together. Add garlic, salt, and pepper. Taste and adjust seasonings.

3. Pour over pasta. Add all vegetables. Toss gently.

4. Let flavors blend at room temperature for at least one hour. Serve over greens.

Exchanges/Choices		
3 Starch	Calories 405	Potassium 355 mg
1 Vegetable	Calories from Fat 145	Total Carbohydrate 55 g
2 1/2 Fat	Total Fat 16.0 g	Dietary Fiber 5 g
	Saturated Fat 2.0 g	Sugars 3 g
	Trans Fat 0.0 g	Protein 11 g
	Cholesterol 0 mg	Phosphorus 145 mg
	Sodium 300 mg	

Fennel, Radicchio & Orange Salad

SERVES: 4 / SERVING SIZE: 1/4 RECIPE

The sweet flavor of the orange offsets the bitter radicchio and complements the licorice flavor of the fennel.

» 1 small head green leaf lettuce or baby spinach, torn into bite-size pieces
» 1 small head radicchio, torn into bite sized pieces
» 1 small bupound fennel, thinly sliced in rounds and cut in half
» 1/4 cup toasted pignoli nuts (pine nuts)
» 1 11-ounce can Mandarin oranges, drained
» 2 tablespoons extra virgin olive oil
» 1 tablespoon white balsamic vinegar
» 1/2 teaspoon fine sea salt
» 1/4 teaspoon freshly ground black pepper

1. Mix all ingredients together and serve immediately.

Exchanges/Choices	Calories 155	Potassium 365 mg
1/2 Fruit	Calories from Fat 115	Total Carbohydrate 10 g
1 Vegetable	Total Fat 13.0 g	Dietary Fiber 2 g
2 1/2 Fat	Saturated Fat 1.4 g	Sugars 6 g
	Trans Fat 0.0 g	Protein 3 g
	Cholesterol 0 mg	Phosphorus 90 mg
	Sodium 325 mg	

Black-Eyed Peas and Orange Salad

SERVES: 4 / SERVING SIZE: 1/4 RECIPE

Also known as cowpeas, black-eyed peas are rich in fiber, potassium, protein, and iron, but low in fat and sodium.

» 1 tablespoon canola oil
» 2 cloves garlic, minced
» 1 cup shredded red cabbage
» 4 cups baby spinach
» 15 ounces canned black-eyed peas, drained
» 2 navel oranges, peeled, halved, and sliced 1/4-inch thick
» 1 tablespoon raspberry vinegar
» 1 medium sweet onion, shaved
» 1/2 cup walnuts, chopped

1. Thinly film a large sauté pan with canola oil and heat to medium.

2. Add garlic and cabbage and sauté until cabbage begins to wilt. Add spinach and wilt slightly.

3. Divide spinach and cabbage between four dinner plates. Top with a spoonful of black-eyed peas and orange slices.

4. Sprinkle with raspberry vinegar. Sprinkle shaved onion and walnuts on top.

Exchanges/Choices	Calories 300	Potassium 865 mg
1 Starch	Calories from Fat 125	Total Carbohydrate 38g
1/2 Fruit	Total Fat 14.0 g	Dietary Fiber 10 g
2 Vegetable 1	Saturated Fat 1.3 g	Sugars 16 g
Lean Meat	Trans Fat 0.0 g	Protein 11 g
2 Fat	Cholesterol 0 mg	Phosphorus 230 mg
	Sodium 175 mg	

CHAPTER 4:
Soups, Stews & Chilis

The Stress Free Diabetes Kitchen

Soups, Stews & Chilis

Tuscan-Style White Bean Soup

SERVES: 12 / SERVING SIZE: 1/12 RECIPE

This soup was inspired by one of my many trips to Italy. You will find delicious white bean soups all over Italy. This one was inspired by the soup we enjoyed in Tuscany.

» 1 tablespoon extra virgin olive oil
» 2 cups diced onion
» 4 large garlic cloves, minced
» 1 cup carrot, cut into 1/2-inch thick slices
» 1 cup celery, cut into 1/2-inch thick slices
» 2 teaspoons dried marjoram (or oregano)
» 2 teaspoons dried basil
» 4 cups small white beans, dried and soaked overnight, or 3 (15-ounce) cans, drained and rinsed well
» 2–2 1/2 quarts low-sodium chicken stock
» 2 bay leaves
» 1 teaspoon fine sea salt
» 4 or 5 turns of freshly ground pepper
» 8 cups chopped Tuscan kale or baby spinach
» Parmigiano-Reggiano (optional, for garnish)

1. Thinly film a soup pot with oil. Add onion and cook until browned. Add garlic, carrots, and celery. Cook until celery begins to soften, approximately 2–3 minutes. Pinch marjoram and basil between your fingers and rub to release oils. Let herbs fall into soup. Mix well and cook 2 additional minutes.

2. Add beans, stock, and bay leaves. Season with salt and pepper. Cook at least 1 hour. Add chopped kale and cook another 20–30 minutes, or until kale is tender.

COOK'S TIP:
This soup will thicken if allowed to cook several hours. It can be made a day or two ahead. When making soup with dried beans, it will take longer for the soup to thicken.

Exchanges/Choices
2 1/2 Starch
1 Vegetable
1 Lean Meat

Calories 270
  Calories from Fat 20
Total Fat 2.0 g
  Saturated Fat 0.5 g
  Trans Fat 0.0 g
Cholesterol 5 mg
Sodium 310 mg

Potassium 1340 mg
Total Carbohydrate 47 g
  Dietary Fiber 12 g
  Sugars 6 g
Protein 19 g
Phosphorus 235 mg

Courmayeur Soup

SERVES: 8 / SERVING SIZE: 1/8 RECIPE

This soup is reminiscent of a wonderful dish I had in Courmayeur, Italy in the Italian Alps. The dish is traditionally called Zuppe Valpellinentze.

» 3/4 pound Italian sausage, turkey, or chicken
» 2 tablespoons extra virgin olive oil
» 1 cup finely diced onion
» 2 cloves garlic, minced
» 8 cups shredded cabbage
» 8 cups low-sodium chicken stock
» 4 thick slices of whole-grain bread, toasted until crispy
» 1 1/2 cups coarsely shredded Asiago Fresco

1. Remove casing from sausage and break up into small pieces. Set aside.

2. Place olive oil, onion, and garlic in medium soup pot. Sauté until onion becomes translucent, about 3 minutes. Add sausage and cook until it begins to brown. Add cabbage. Mix well. Cook 3 minutes until cabbage begins to soften. Add stock. Simmer 15 minutes.

3. Place bread in ovenproof soup bowls or small pie plates. Add soup and top with cheese. Bake in a 425°F oven for 8–10 minutes, or until cheese is golden brown. Serve immediately.

COOK'S TIP:
You can use sweet or hot Italian sausage. If your sausage is spicy, it will provide all the seasonings you need for the soup.

Exchanges
1/2 Starch
2 Vegetable
1 Med-Fat Meat
1 Fat

Calories 215
   Calories from Fat 90
Total Fat 10.0 g
   Saturated Fat 3.7 g
   Trans Fat 0.1 g
Cholesterol 40 mg
Sodium 470 mg

Potassium 485 mg
Total Carbohydrate 17 g
   Dietary Fiber 4 g
   Sugars 4 g
Protein 14 g
Phosphorus 230 mg

Roasted Pumpkin & Butternut Squash Soup

SERVES: 8 / SERVING SIZE: 1/8 RECIPE

Grocery stores now carry cut Butternut squash, which makes this dish even more "Stress Free." If you want to use cut up Butternut squash, you can use 5 pounds and eliminate the pumpkin. You can even serve this soup in a pumpkin for a special occasion.

» 1 butternut squash, about 2 1/2 pounds, cut into large chunks
» 1 pumpkin, about 2 1/2 pounds, cut into large chunks
» 6 cups low-sodium vegetable or chicken stock
» 2 tablespoons finely minced ginger
» 1 cup evaporated skim milk, well shaken
» 1 teaspoon ground nutmeg
» 1/2 teaspoon ground cinnamon
» Fine sea salt to taste
» Freshly ground black pepper to taste

{ COOK'S TIP:
Can be made a day or two ahead. Good source of fiber. }

1. Preheat oven to 400°F. Roast squash and pumpkin on parchment-lined baking sheet until tender. (This can take anywhere from 30 minutes to one hour.) Cool.

2. Scrape flesh from skin and place in food processor. Add some stock to make a smooth consistency and purée.

3. Place squash and pumpkin in large saucepan and add remaining ingredients. Bring to boil and reduce to simmer. Cook 20–30 minutes to allow flavors to blend.

4. Adjust seasonings before serving. Garnish with a dollop of non-fat sour cream, a drizzle of pumpkin seed oil, and pumpkin, squash, or sunflower seeds.

Exchanges/Choices		
1 Starch		
	Calories 90	Potassium 605 mg
	Calories from Fat 0	Total Carbohydrate 19g
	Total Fat 0.0 g	Dietary Fiber 4 g
	Saturated Fat 0.2 g	Sugars 7 g
	Trans Fat 0.0 g	Protein 4 g
	Cholesterol 0 mg	Phosphorus 145 mg
	Sodium 145 mg	

Mushroom Soup

SERVES: 8 / SERVING SIZE: 1/8 RECIPE

To make this creamier, you can purée the soup with a stick blender. I like it with some chunks of mushroom and onion, so I typically purée only half of it.

» 20 ounces mushrooms, such as portobello or cremini
» 2 tablespoons extra virgin olive oil
» 2 large sweet onions, thinly sliced
» 4 cloves garlic, minced
» 32 ounces low-sodium mushroom, chicken, or vegetable stock
» 1/2 teaspoon fine sea salt
» 1/4 teaspoon freshly cracked black pepper
» 1/2 cup chopped herbs, such as parsley and basil (plus additional for garnish)

1. Slice or chop mushrooms into bite-size pieces. Place olive oil and onions in pan. Cook until onions are translucent. Add garlic and cook until fragrant.

2. Add mushrooms to pan. Cook 3–5 minutes until moisture is released. Add stock, salt, and pepper and cook 20 minutes. Add 1/2 cup fresh herbs and cook 5 minutes more.

3. Garnish with any additional fresh herbs you desire. Serve.

Exchanges/Choices		
2 Vegetable	Calories 85	Potassium 520 mg
1/2 Fat	Calories from Fat 30	Total Carbohydrate 10 g
	Total Fat 3.5 g	Dietary Fiber 1 g
	Saturated Fat 0.6 g	Sugars 6 g
	Trans Fat 0.0 g	Protein 4 g
	Cholesterol 0 mg	Phosphorus 125 mg
	Sodium 200 mg	

Tomato Mushroom Soup

SERVES: 8 / SERVING SIZE: 1/8 RECIPE

» 1 tablespoon extra virgin olive oil
» 2 large sweet onions, thinly sliced
» 1 clove garlic, minced
» 2 teaspoons Italian seasoning blend
» 1 medium potato, shredded
» 20 ounces mushrooms, such as portobel-
   loor cremini, chopped into bite-size
   pieces
» 15 ounces canned, diced tomatoes
» 32 ounces low-sodium chicken or vegetable stock
» Fresh chopped herbs (optional)
» Parmigiano-Reggiano (optional)

1. Place olive oil in large soup pan. Add onions, garlic, and Italian seasoning blend and cook until onions begin to turn golden brown. Add pota- toes and cook until potatoes begin to soften. Add mushrooms and sauté for 2 minutes. Add tomatoes and stock and bring to a boil. Turn down heat and simmer for 30 minutes.

2. Serve with fresh herbs and grated Parmigiano-Reg- giano, if desired.

Exchanges/Choices	Calories 95	Potassium 680 mg
3 Vegetable	Calories from Fat 20	Total Carbohydrate 16 g
1/2 Fat	Total Fat 2.0 g	Dietary Fiber 2 g
	Saturated Fat 0.4 g	Sugars 7 g
	Trans Fat 0.0 g	Protein 4 g
	Cholesterol 0 mg	Phosphorus 150 mg
	Sodium 130 mg	

Spicy Vegetable, Bean, and Egg Drop Soup

SERVES: 8 / SERVING SIZE: 1/8 RECIPE

This soup is wonderful on its own, but when you add the egg and poach it in the soup, the soup becomes rich and creamy while still maintaining the health and nutritional value of vegetable bean soup.

» 2 tablespoons extra virgin olive oil
» 1 medium onion, diced
» 4 large garlic cloves, minced
» 1 cup carrot, cut into 1/2-inch thick slices
» 1 cup celery, cut into 1/2-inch thick slices
» 2 teaspoons Italian seasoning blend
» 2 (16-ounce) cans pinto beans (or your favorite variety), drained and rinsed
» 1 cup frozen corn
» 1 cup frozen lima beans
» 10 ounces frozen, chopped spinach
» 15 ounces diced tomatoes with green chilies
» 28 ounces crushed tomatoes
» 15 ounces low-sodium vegetable or chicken stock
» 8 large eggs

1. Place oil in soup pot. Add onion and cook on medium-high heat until it begins to brown. Add garlic, carrots, and celery. Cook until celery begins to soften, approximately 2–3 minutes. Pinch Italian seasoning blend between your fingers and rub to release oils. Let herbs fall into soup. Mix well and cook 2 minutes.

2. Add beans, corn, lima beans, spinach, both kinds of tomatoes, and stock. Cook 30 minutes or longer.

3. Crack the eggs into a small bowl and drop them into the soup pan one at a time. Cover and let the eggs poach on top of the soup. This will take 3–5 minutes. Serve the soup in large bowl with the poached egg in the center.

Exchanges/Choices
1 1/2 Starch
3 Vegetable
1 Med-Fat Meat
1/2 Fat

Calories 300
   Calories from Fat 80
Total Fat 9.0 g
   Saturated Fat 2.3 g
   Trans Fat 0.0 g
Cholesterol 185 mg
Sodium 640 mg

Potassium 1025 mg
Total Carbohydrate 40 g
   Dietary Fiber 12 g
   Sugars 9 g
Protein 17 g
Phosphorus 305 mg

Spinach, Mushroom, and Tortellini Soup

SERVES: 6 / SERVING SIZE: 1/6 RECIPE

This soup goes a long way because of the tortellini. You can serve it as a first course or a whole meal and it is great as a "leftover."

» 1 tablespoon extra virgin olive oil
» 2 cloves garlic, minced
» 32 ounces low-sodium chicken stock
» 32 ounces low-sodium vegetable stock (or use all chicken stock)
» 28 ounces diced tomatoes (canned or fresh)
» 12 ounces water
» 1 cup fresh basil, chopped
» 1/2 cup fresh oregano, roughly chopped
» 2 cups baby spinach
» 10 ounces cheese tortellini (or plain pasta if you prefer)
» 10 ounces sliced fresh cremini mushrooms (optional)
» Parmigiano-Reggiano (optional)

1. Heat olive oil and garlic in soup pot over medium heat until garlic is fragrant.

2. Add stocks, tomatoes, and water. Bring to a boil.

3. Add basil, oregano, spinach, tortellini, and mushrooms. Cook until tortellini is done, approximately 10 minutes. More water or stock can be added to achieve desired consistency.

4. Garnish with Parmigiano-Reggiano, if desired. Serve.

Exchanges/Choices		
1 1/2 Starch	Calories 225	Potassium 580 mg
2 Vegetable	Calories from Fat 65	Total Carbohydrate 30 g
1 Fat	Total Fat 7.0 g	Dietary Fiber 5 g
	Saturated Fat 1.8 g	Sugars 5 g
	Trans Fat 0.0 g	Protein 11 g
	Cholesterol 20 mg	Phosphorus 90 mg
	Sodium 560 mg	

Lemon Chicken Soup (Avgolemono)

SERVES: 8 / SERVING SIZE: 1/8 RECIPE

This soup is a traditional Greek dish that can be prepared in almost no time if you have leftover roast chicken.

Chicken Soup

» 3–4 pound roasting chicken
» 2 –2 1/2 quarts of water
» 1 teaspoon whole black peppercorns
» Salt to taste
» 1 medium carrot, cut into large chunks
» 1 medium onion, cut into large chunks
» 1 stalk celery, cut into large chunks
» 1 cup uncooked orzo (rice-shaped pasta)

Avgolemono

» 2 large eggs
» 3 tablespoons fresh lemon juice

1. Place chicken in an 8-quart soup pot with water to cover. Add peppercorns, salt, carrot, onion, and celery. Bring to boil, cover, and simmer for 2 hours or until chicken is tender. Adjust salt to taste.

2. Remove chicken and set aside. Strain chicken stock and skim any visible fat. Add orzo, cover, and simmer until orzo is tender, approximately 15–20 minutes.

3. While orzo is cooking, chop chicken into bite-size pieces.

4. Beat eggs well and gradually beat in lemon juice either by hand or with a food processor. Add 2 cups broth slowly and beat constantly until well blended and thickened.

5. Combine sauce, cooked chicken, and remaining broth. Serve.

Exchanges/Choices		
1 Starch	Calories 265	Potassium 355 mg
3 Lean Meat	Calories from Fat 80	Total Carbohydrate 19 g
1 Fat	Total Fat 9.0 g	Dietary Fiber 1 g
	Saturated Fat 2.5 g	Sugars 3 g
	Trans Fat 0.0 g	Protein 25 g
	Cholesterol 100 mg	Phosphorus 210 mg
	Sodium 155 mg	

Cream of Asparagus Soup

SERVES: 4 / SERVING SIZE: 1/4 RECIPE

There are many tricks to making a creamed soup. You can either purée the ingredients in a blender or garnish your soup with a healthy, rich, creamy ingredient like part-skim ricotta and stir it into your soup.

» 3 pounds fresh asparagus, cut into 1-inch pieces
» 1 large Yukon Gold potato, cut into large chunks (about 2 inches square)
» 6 cups low-sodium chicken or vegetable stock
» 3 whole garlic cloves
» Fine sea salt
» Freshly ground pepper
» 2 bay leaves
» 1 cup fresh ricotta cheese
» Whole nutmeg

1. Cook asparagus, potato, stock, garlic, salt, a few grinds of black pepper, and bay leaves in a large soup pot for approximately 20 minutes. Remove bay leaves.

2. Place in food processor and pulse until smooth. Adjust salt and pepper to taste.

3. Serve with a dollop of ricotta cheese and a fresh grinding of nutmeg.

Exchanges/Choices	Calories 205	Potassium 990 mg
1 Starch	Calories from Fat 55	Total Carbohydrate 25 g
2 Vegetable	Total Fat 6.0 g	Dietary Fiber 5 g
1 Med-Fat Meat	Saturated Fat 3.4 g	Sugars 4 g
	Trans Fat 0.0 g	Protein 16 g
	Cholesterol 25 mg	Phosphorus 310 mg
	Sodium 235 mg	

Minestrone Soup (Italian Vegetable, Bean, and Pasta Soup)

SERVES: 10 / SERVING SIZE: 1/10 RECIPE

Minestrone means "big soup" in Italian. It is usually considered a whole meal. Serve with a sprinkle of freshly grated Parmigiano-Reggiano, a mixed green salad, and crusty bread for a satisfying meal.

» 1 tablespoon extra virgin olive oil
» 2 cups chopped onion
» 6 large cloves garlic, minced
» 1 1/2 cups celery, sliced
» 1 1/2 cups sliced carrots
» 2 cups zucchini, quartered, thinly sliced
» 2 cups peeled and diced eggplant
» 56 ounces canned, diced tomatoes
» 4 cups low-sodium chicken or vegetable stock
» 6 cups water
» 2 15-ounce cans small white beans or chick-peas, drained and rinsed well

» 1 1/2 cups uncooked small pasta, such as orzo, Ditalini, or Acini di pepe
» 1 cup fresh basil, roughly chopped
» 1/2 cup fresh oregano, finely chopped
» 4 bay leaves
» 3/4 teaspoon fine sea salt
» Freshly ground pepper to taste
» 1 teaspoon Parmigiano-Reggiano, grated (optional)

(Continued on next page)

Exchanges/Choices		
2 Starch	Calories 260	Potassium 880 mg
3 Vegetable	Calories from Fat 25	Total Carbohydrate 50 g
1/2 Fat	Total Fat 3.0 g	Dietary Fiber 11 g
	Saturated Fat 0.5 g	Sugars 11 g
	Trans Fat 0.0 g	Protein 11 g
	Cholesterol 0 mg	Phosphorus 190 mg
	Sodium 570 mg	

(Minestrone Soup Continued)

1. Thinly film a soup pot with olive oil. Add onion and cook until it begins to brown. Add garlic, celery, and carrots. Sauté 3–5 minutes. (Don't let garlic get to the dark brown or black stage.)

2. Add zucchini, eggplant, tomatoes, stock, water, and beans. Cook until vegetables are tender, 10–15 minutes.

3. Add pasta, herbs, salt, and a few grindings of pepper. Cook until pasta is al dente, approximately 10–15 minutes. Remove bay leaves before serving. Sprinkle with Parmigiano-Reggiano, if desired.

COOK'S TIP:
» Remove the bay leaves before serving. They are sharp and can cause injury if swallowed.
» Rinsing the beans also eliminates any unpleasant gasses.

Cream of Broccoli & Garlic Soup with Asiago & Speck

SERVES: 6 / SERVING SIZE: 1/6 RECIPE

Speck is dry, cured, boldly seasoned ham from the North of Italy. It is well seasoned when purchased, so you generally don't have to add a lot of additional seasoning to the dish. This means less work for you. You can purchase already diced speck in the grocery store.

» 1 head broccoli
» 2 large cloves garlic
» 1 medium onion
» 1 Yukon Gold potato, (weighing approximately 8 ounces)
» 1 tablespoon extra virgin olive oil
» 4 cups low-sodium chicken or vegetable stock
» 4 ounces finely diced speck
» Freshly ground black pepper, to taste
» 1/2 cup coarsely grated Asiago Fresca

1. Cut broccoli into small florets. Crush the garlic with the sides of a chef's knife and discard the skins. Peel and roughly chop onion. Peel and grate potato.

2. Place olive oil in large soup pan. Add broccoli, garlic, onion, and potato. Sauté until garlic becomes fragrant.

3. Add stock to pot. Bring to a boil, turn down to a simmer, and cook for 10 minutes or until broccoli is soft and tender.

4. Using an immersion blender; purée until smooth. Add speck and simmer another 10 minutes. Add a few grinds of freshly ground black pepper. Taste and adjust seasonings.

5. Ladle into bowls and garnish with cheese.

Exchanges/Choices		
1/2 Starch	Calories 175	Potassium 590 mg
1 Vegetable	Calories from Fat 70	Total Carbohydrate 14 g
1 Med-Fat Meat	Total Fat 8.0 g	Dietary Fiber 3 g
1/2 Fat	Saturated Fat 3.2 g	Sugars 3 g
	Trans Fat 0.0 g	Protein 12 g
	Cholesterol 25 mg	Phosphorus 210 mg
	Sodium 495 mg	

Tomato & Roasted Garlic Soup with Gorgonzola Crouton

SERVES: 8 / SERVING SIZE: 1/8 RECIPE

» 18 fresh plum tomatoes, peeled and chopped, or 2 28-ounce cans diced tomatoes
» 1/2 teaspoon fine sea salt
» Freshly ground pepper
» 1 tablespoon extra virgin olive oil
» 2 tablespoons Roasted Garlic (page 15)
» 1 cup fresh basil leaves, torn just before adding to the soup
» 8 slices (1/2 ounce each) multi-grain Italian bread or baguette
» Olive oil spray
» 2 1/2 ounces crumbled Gorgonzola cheese

1. Mix tomatoes, salt, and pepper in a medium or large bowl.

2. Place a 4-quart saucepan on burner and add olive oil and tomatoes.

3. Cook until tomatoes fall apart. Purée with stick blender of run through food processor. Add Roasted Garlic (page 15) and simmer. Tear basil leaves and add to tomato mixture.

4. Lightly spray both sides of each slice of bread with olive oil spray. Grill or broil until golden. Place 1 tablespoon Gorgonzola on each piece of toasted bread. Broil until cheese starts to melt.

5. Ladle soup into bowl and top with bread and additional basil, if desired.

Exchanges/Choices	Calories 140	Potassium 545 mg
1/2 Starch	Calories from Fat 55	Total Carbohydrate 17 g
2 Vegetable	Total Fat 6.0 g	Dietary Fiber 4 g
1 Fat	Saturated Fat 2.2 g	Sugars 6 g
	Trans Fat 0.1 g	Protein 6 g
	Cholesterol 5 mg	Phosphorus 125 mg
	Sodium 390 mg	

Hot & Sour Soup

SERVES: 4 / SERVING SIZE: 1/4 RECIPE

» 6 cups low-sodium chicken stock
» 1/4 pound lean pork, julienne
» 1 tablespoon Asian garlic chile paste
» 2 tablespoons light soy sauce
» 1 cup shiitake mushrooms, sliced and stems removed
» 1 cup straw mushrooms
» 3/4 teaspoon white pepper, ground
» 1/4 cup white vinegar
» 1/2 cup bamboo shoots, julienned
» 1/2 cup water chestnuts, sliced
» 1/4 cup dried mushrooms, soaked for 1 hour
» 1 12-ounce package cake tofu, 1/4-inch dice
» 5 tablespoons cornstarch
» 5 tablespoons water
» 4 eggs, beaten
» 1 teaspoon sesame oil
» 2–3 thin scallions finely chopped (for garnish)

1. Bring chicken stock to a simmer in a large stock-pot. Add pork, garlic chile paste, soy sauce, and mushrooms. Simmer for 10 minutes. Add pepper, vinegar, bamboo shots, water chestnuts, fungus, and tofu. Simmer for 5 minutes.

2. Mix cornstarch with 5 tablespoons of water and add to the soup.

3. Bring mixture back to a simmer and pour eggs in a very thin stream over the surface. Let stand for 10 seconds before stirring in the sesame oil.

4. Garnish with chopped scallions and serve.

Exchanges/Choices
1/2 Starch
2 Vegetable
2 Med-Fat Meat
1/2 Fat

Calories 280
    Calories from Fat 110
Total Fat 12.0 g
    Saturated Fat 3.4 g
    Trans Fat 0.0 g
Cholesterol 205 mg
Sodium 535 mg

Potassium 830 mg
Total Carbohydrate 18 g
    Dietary Fiber 3 g
    Sugars 2 g
Protein 25 g
Phosphorus 345 mg

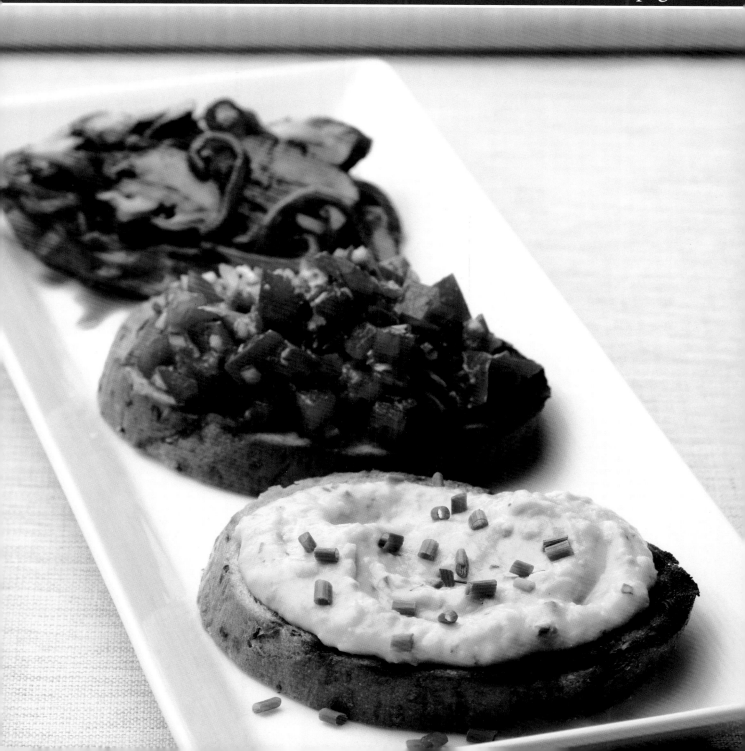

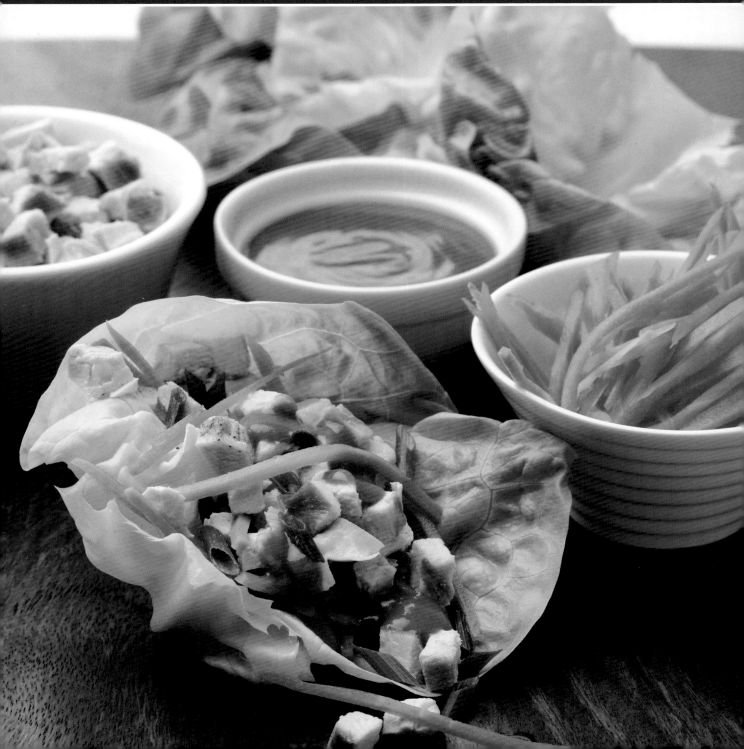

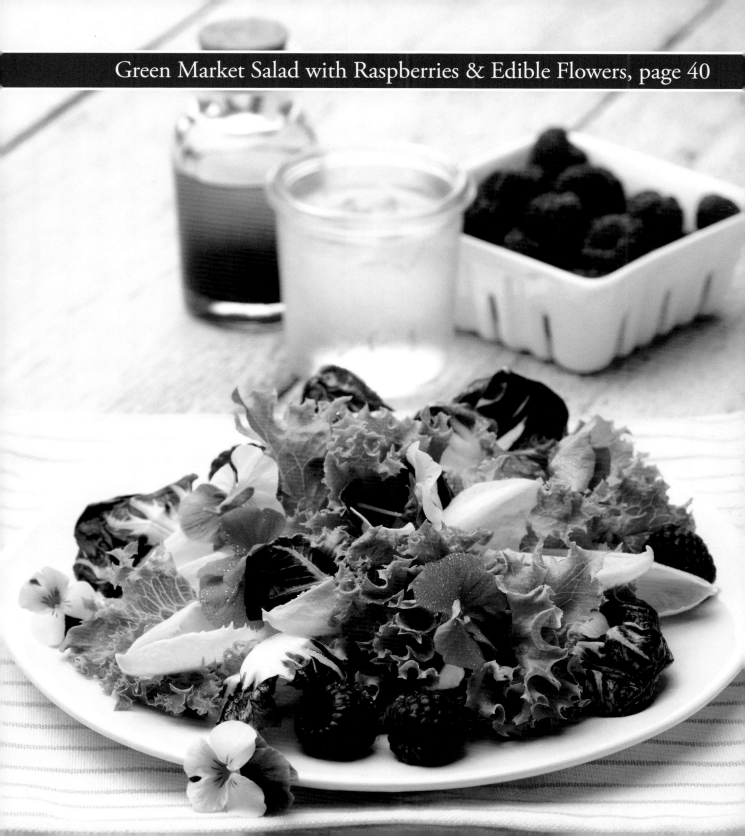

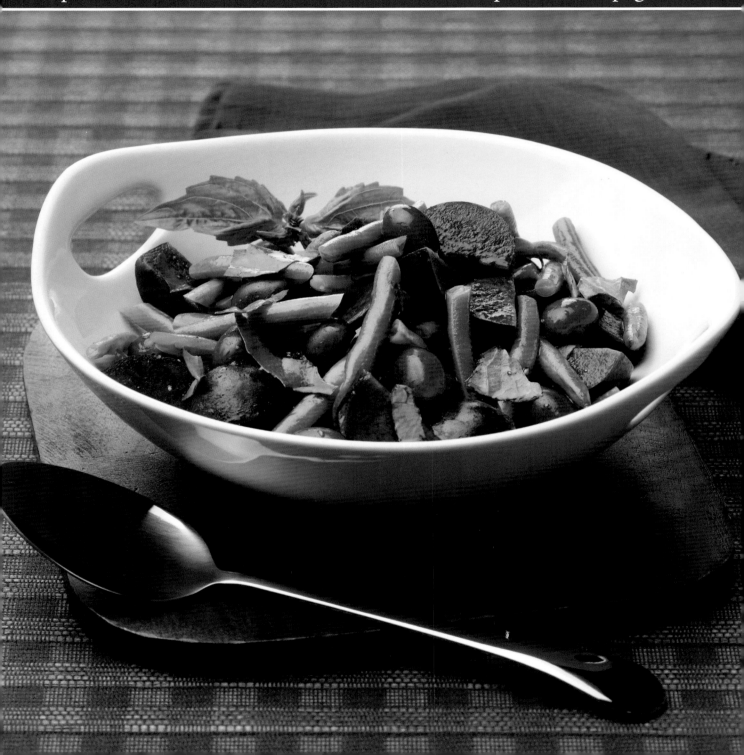

Purple Potato Salad with Green Beans & Tear Drop Tomatoes, page 120

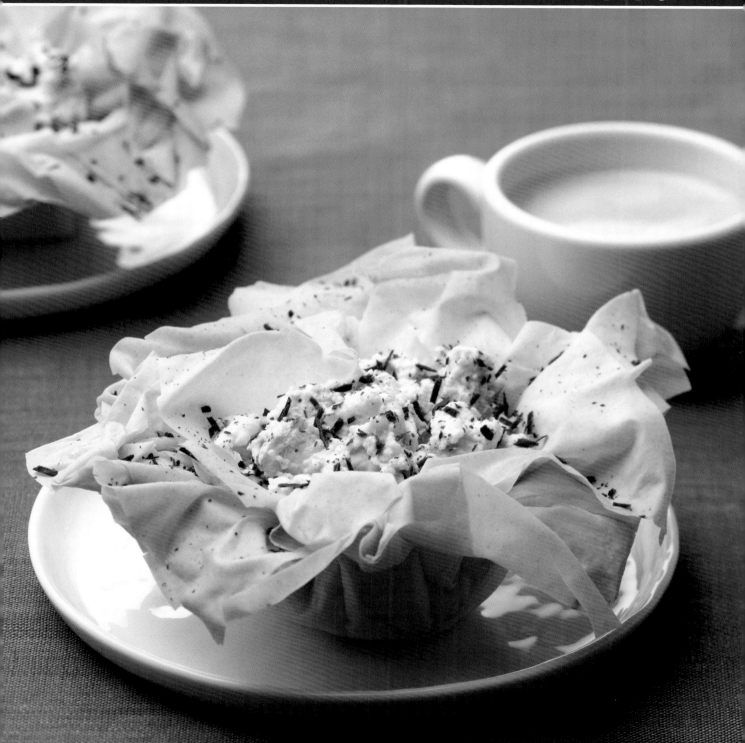

Cannoli Cups, page 181

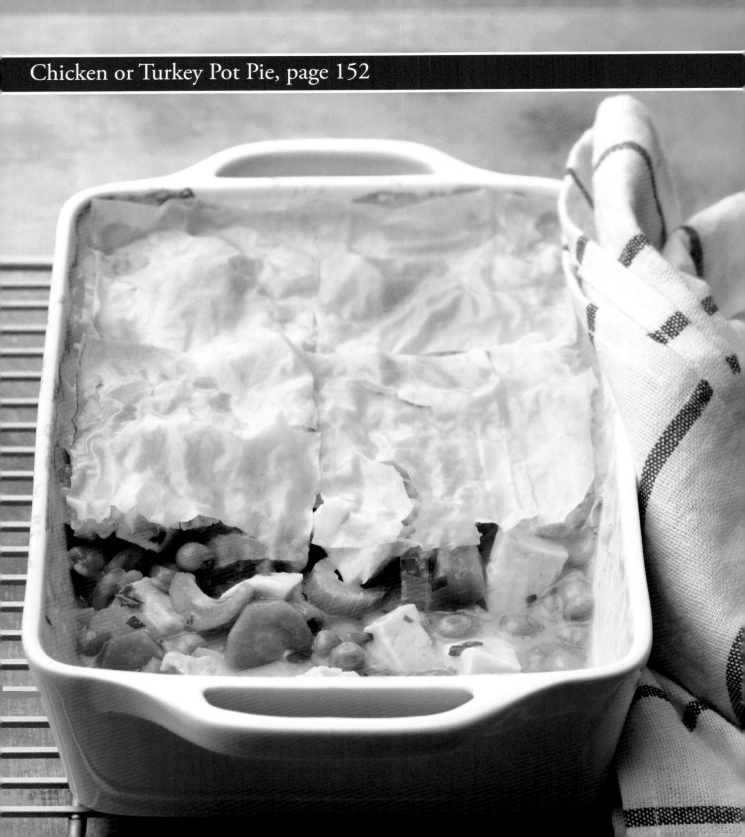

Chicken or Turkey Pot Pie, page 152

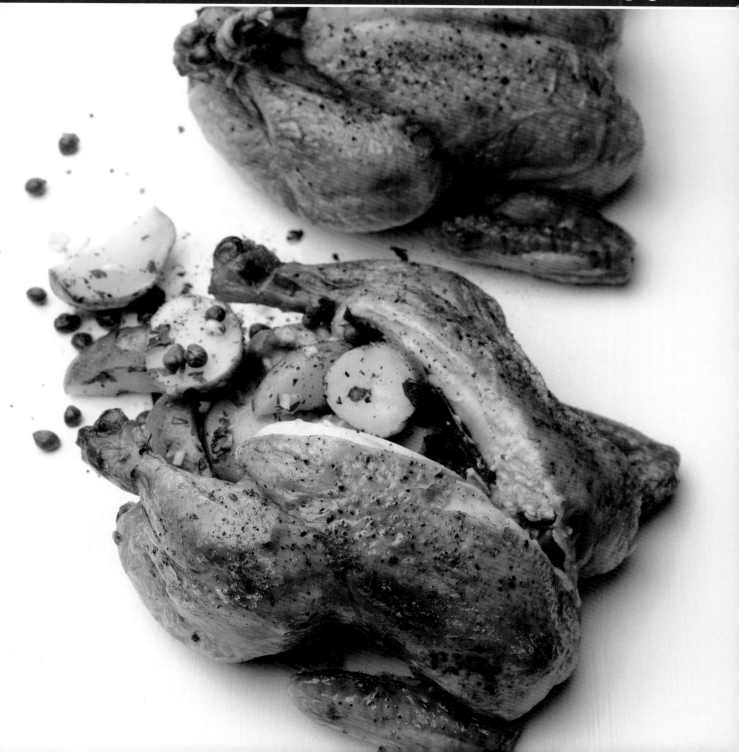

Cornish Hens Stuffed with Potatoes, Capers, and Garlic, page 147

Fresh Picked Apple Crunch Cake, page 183

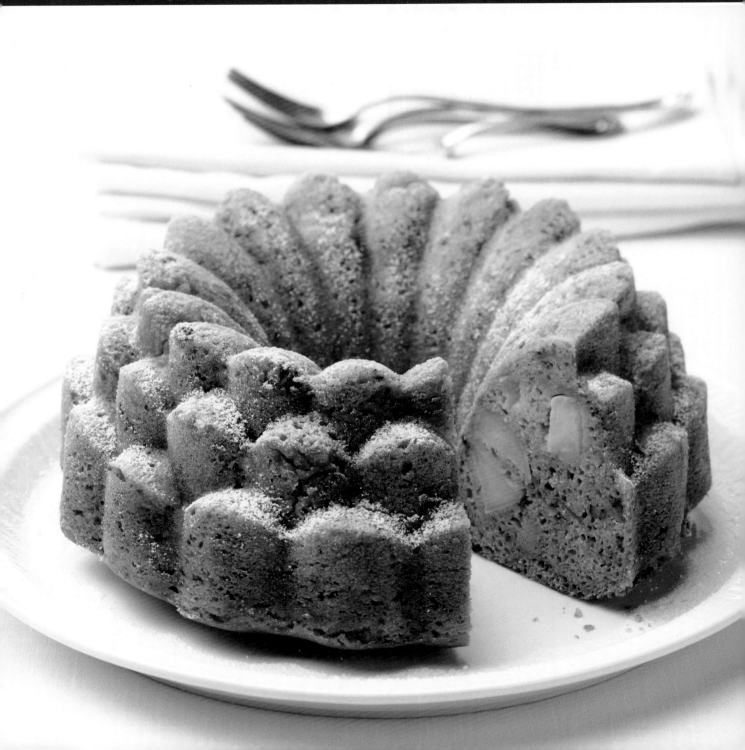

Fresh Vegetable Soup

SERVES: 8 / SERVING SIZE: 1/8 RECIPE

» 1 tablespoon extra virgin olive oil
» 1 cup diced Vidalia or Spanish onion
» 2 large cloves garlic, crushed and peeled
» 3 large carrots, halved lengthwise and
   sliced thinly
» 3 celery ribs, sliced thinly
» 1 large zucchini, quartered and sliced
   thinly
» 1 large yellow squash, quartered and
   sliced thinly
» 10 ounces fresh mushrooms, sliced
» 4 cups low-sodium, vegetable, chicken, or
   mushroom stock
» 1/2 cup chopped fresh basil
» 2 tablespoons minced fresh oregano
» 1 teaspoon fine sea salt
» 1/2 teaspoon freshly ground pepper

1. Place olive oil in soup pot. Add onions and cook until they begin to brown. Add garlic, carrots, and celery and cook 5–10 minutes until vegetables are soft.

2. Add zucchini, squash, mushrooms, and stock. Cook another 20 minutes.

3. Add basil, oregano, salt and pepper. Cook 5 minutes more. Adjust consistency by adding additional stock, if desired. Serve with additional fresh herbs as garnish.

Exchanges/Choices		
2 Vegetable	Calories 70	Potassium 545 mg
1/2 Fat	Calories from Fat 20	Total Carbohydrate 11 g
	Total Fat 2.0 g	Dietary Fiber 3 g
	Saturated Fat 0.3 g	Sugars 5 g
	Trans Fat 0.0 g	Protein 3 g
	Cholesterol 0 mg	Phosphorus 105 mg
	Sodium 410 mg	

Black Bean Soup with Cilantro Cream

SERVES 6: / SERVING SIZE: 1/6 RECIPE

This soup can be made from basic ingredients in your pantry.

» 1 bunch cilantro or flat Italian parsley
» 6 ounces plain, nonfat yogurt
» 1 tablespoon extra virgin olive oil
» 1 large Spanish onion, chopped
» 4 carrots, sliced
» 4 stalks celery, sliced
» 3 cloves garlic, minced
» 3 bay leaves
» 1/2 cup fresh basil, chopped
» 1 tablespoon dried oregano
» 2 15-ounce cans black beans, drained and rinsed
» 1 15-ounce can diced tomatoes
» 32 ounce low-sodium chicken or vegetable stock

1. Mix two tablespoons minced cilantro with plain, low-fat yogurt. Drain through yogurt strainer (in fridge) while soup is cooking.

2. Add olive oil to stockpot. Heat oil and add onions, carrots, and celery. Cook 5 minutes. Add garlic and herbs. Cook until fragrant.

3. Add beans, tomatoes, and stock to pot. Simmer 20–30 minutes.

4. Garnish soup with cilantro cream or parsley, if desired. Serve.

COOK'S TIP:

Make your own yogurt strainer by placing a coffee filter in a small colander and then place in a large bowl.

Exchanges/Choices
1 Starch
3 Vegetable
1 Lean Meat
1/2 Fat

Calories 210
   Calories from Fat 30
Total Fat 3.5 g
   Saturated Fat 0.9 g
   Trans Fat 0.0 g
Cholesterol 5 mg
Sodium 340 mg

Potassium 990 mg
Total Carbohydrate 34 g
   Dietary Fiber 11 g
   Sugars 9 g
Protein 12 g
Phosphorus 225 mg

Cream of Potato & Garlic Soup

SERVES: 6 / SERVING SIZE: 1/6 RECIPE

» 3 pounds Yukon Gold potatoes, peeled and cut into 1-inch chunks
» 3 whole garlic cloves
» Fine sea salt
» Freshly ground pepper
» 2 bay leaves
» 3 cups low-sodium chicken or vegetable stock

1. Add potatoes, garlic, salt, a few grinds of black pepper, bay leaves, and stock to large stockpot and cook over high heat until potatoes are fork tender, approximately 20 minutes.

2. Remove bay leaves. Place soup in food processor and pulse until smooth.

3. Adjust salt and pepper to taste. Serve.

Exchanges/Choices		
2 1/2 Starch		

Calories 160		Potassium 675 mg
Calories from Fat 0		Total Carbohydrate 36 g
Total Fat 0.0 g		Dietary Fiber 3 g
Saturated Fat 0.1 g		Sugars 2 g
Trans Fat 0.0 g		Protein 4 g
Cholesterol 0 mg		Phosphorus 90 mg
Sodium 55 mg		

Chicken Pumpkin Chili

SERVES: 8 / SERVING SIZE: 1/8 RECIPE

» 1 tablespoon extra virgin olive oil
» 2 cups chopped onion
» 2 cups chopped red bell pepper
» 2 garlic cloves, crushed
» 12 ounces beer
» 1 cup low-fat, low-sodium chicken stock
» 3 tablespoons chili powder
» 1/2 teaspoon fine sea salt
» 1 28-ounce can plum tomatoes
» 1 1/2 pounds boneless, skinless chicken breast, cut into cubes
» 2 cups cubed fresh pumpkin, cooked
» 2 tablespoons chopped fresh cilantro
» 1 15-ounce can small white or pink beans, rinsed and drained

1. Heat oil in large saucepan over medium heat. Add onion and sauté until lightly browned. Add bell pepper and garlic, sauté until peppers begin to soften, about 3 minutes.

2. Add beer, stock, chili powder, salt, tomatoes, and chicken. Bring to boil and quickly reduce to simmer. Cook 20 minutes or until chicken is done.

3. Stir in pumpkin, cilantro, and beans, cook 5 minutes.

4. Optional garnishes for this recipe are toasted pumpkin seeds, low-fat cheddar cheese, Jalapeño peppers, or non-fat sour cream or yogurt.

{ COOK'S TIP:
To toast pumpkin seeds: Remove the seeds from the pumpkin. Scrape as much as possible, but do not rinse. Spread on a cookie sheet and bake at 300°F for 45 minutes. }

Exchanges/Choices
1 Starch
2 Vegetable
2 Lean Meat
1/2 Fat

Calories 240
  Calories from Fat 45
Total Fat 5.0 g
  Saturated Fat 1.0 g
  Trans Fat 0.0 g
Cholesterol 50 mg
Sodium 590 mg

Potassium 805 mg
Total Carbohydrate 25 g
  Dietary Fiber 7 g
  Sugars 6 g
Protein 23   g
Phosphorus 250 mg

Mixed Bean Chili

SERVES: 8 / SERVING SIZE: 1/8 RECIPE

» 1 teaspoon canola oil
» 1 large Spanish onion, chopped (1 1/2 cups)
» 2 large green bell peppers, chopped
» 2 celery stalks, sliced 1/2-inch thick
» 2 large carrots, sliced 1/2-inch thick
» 3 garlic cloves, minced
» 1 tablespoon minced jalapeño pepper (optional)
» 2 teaspoons dried oregano
» Pinch cayenne pepper
» 2 teaspoons cumin
» Pinch ground cloves
» 30 ounces canned pink beans (or your favorite beans), drained and rinsed
» 8 cups diced tomatoes
» 1/2 cup fresh chopped cilantro or flat Italian parsley
» 1/3 cup light cheddar cheese, grated (for garnish)
» 1 bunch scallions, sliced (for garnish)

1. Heat the oil in a large soup pot over medium-high heat. Add the onion, peppers, celery, and carrots and sauté until onion is translucent. Stir in the garlic, jalapeño, oregano, cayenne, cumin, and cloves. Sauté another 2–3 minutes.

2. Add the beans, tomatoes, and cilantro and bring to boil. Reduce the heat and simmer covered for 30–60 minutes, or until flavors blend. Adjust seasonings before serving.

3. Ladle into bowls and garnish with cheese and sliced scallions.

{ **COOK'S TIP:**
Wear rubber gloves when seeding and chopping the jalapeño. }

Exchanges/Choices	Calories 180	Total Carbohydrate 33 g
1 Starch	Calories from Fat 20	Dietary Fiber 10 g
3 Vegetable	Total Fat 2.5 g	Sugars 9 g
1/2 Fat	Saturated Fat 0.7 g	Protein 10 g
	Trans Fat 0.0 g	Phosphorus 195 mg
	Cholesterol 0 mg	
	Sodium 185 mg	
	Potassium 980 mg	

Veal Stew

SERVES: 6 / SERVING SIZE: 1/6 RECIPE

» 1 pound veal stew meat (also known as chuck for stew), cut into bite-size pieces
» 1 cup flour (for dredging the meat)
» Fine sea salt
» Freshly ground pepper
» 2 tablespoons extra virgin olive oil
» 1 cup baby carrots, sliced vertically if thick
» 2 cloves garlic, minced
» 1 large sweet potato or Yukon Gold, cut into 1/2–1 inch cubes
» 1/2 cup fresh basil, chopped
» 1 quart low-sodium chicken or veal stock
» 1 cup dry red wine (such as Burgundy or Sangiovese)
» 8 ounces frozen pearl onions
» 8 ounces frozen, cut green beans
» 2 bay leaves

1. Trim meat to get rid of any visible fat. Season the flour with salt and pepper. Toss the meat in the flour to dredge.

2. Heat the stockpot and thinly film the bottom with olive oil.

3. Add the meat and brown well on all sides. Make sure that you don't crowd the pan and cook meat in one single layer at a time. Remove meat as it browns.

4. Add carrots, garlic, and potatoes. Cook 3–5 minutes to brown. Hold basil in between your thumb and forefinger and rub between your fingers before adding to stew. (The heat and the oils in your fingers will release the fragrances in the herb.)

(Continued on next page)

Exchanges/Choices
1 Starch
2 Vegetable
2 Lean Meat
1/2 Fat

Calories 250
   Calories from Fat 65
Total Fat 7.0 g
   Saturated Fat 1.4 g
   Trans Fat 0.0 g
Cholesterol 65 mg
Sodium 150 mg

Potassium 550 mg
Total Carbohydrate 26 g
   Dietary Fiber 4 g
   Sugars 5 g
Protein 20 g
Phosphorus 175 mg

(Veal Stew Continued)

5. Return meat to saucepan and add stock, wine, onions, green beans, and bay leaves. Bring to boil, and immediately turn down to medium-low heat. Check seasonings and adjust salt and pepper to taste.

6. Cook on low at least 1 1/2 hours, so that flavors blend and meat and vegetables become tender. Do not boil the meat; keep it at a low simmer. You could also transfer this to your slow cooker and cook on low for 6–8 hours, or high for 3–4 hours.

7. If a thicker stew is desired, mix in additional stock and flour and whisk into the hot stew. Continue cooking for 10 minutes to thicken.

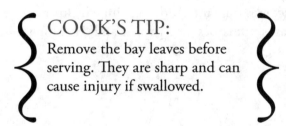

COOK'S TIP:
Remove the bay leaves before serving. They are sharp and can cause injury if swallowed.

Mediterranean Vegetable Stew with Chick Peas

SERVES: 6 / SERVING SIZE: 1/6 RECIPE

If an occasional vegetarian meal is appealing to you, here is a great choice.

» 1 medium eggplant
» 1 medium to large zucchini
» 1/2 teaspoon fine sea salt
» 2 10-ounce cans chick peas, drained and rinsed (or any beans you like)
» 2 tablespoons extra virgin olive oil
» 3 cloves garlic, minced
» 2 teaspoons Italian seasoning blend
» 3 bay leaves
» 28 ounces no-salt-added diced tomatoes
» Freshly ground black pepper

1. Thinly slice zucchini into rounds and set aside. Cut eggplant into similar size pieces. Place eggplant in a bowl and sprinkle with salt. Toss well. (This will help to prevent eggplant from absorbing too much oil.)

2. Drain chickpeas in a colander and rinse well.

3. Place the olive oil in the skillet. Add garlic and eggplant and cook until they begin to soften. Clear a space in the bottom of the pan and add the Italian seasoning. Cook 1 minute until the seasoning becomes fragrant. Add zucchini, chickpeas, bay leaves, tomatoes, and pepper and cook for 10 minutes.

COOK'S TIP:
» Draining canned beans helps to remove preservatives and some of the gas.
» Remove bay leaves before serving. They can cause injury if swallowed.

Exchanges/Choices		
1 Starch	Calories 195	Potassium
2 Vegetable	Calories from Fat 55	615 mg
1 Fat	Total Fat 6.0 g	Total Carbohydrate 30 g
	Saturated Fat 0.9 g	Dietary Fiber 8 g
	Trans Fat 0.0 g	Sugars 9 g
	Cholesterol 0 mg	Protein 7g
	Sodium 350 mg	Phosphorus 145 mg

CHAPTER 5:
Eggs and Egg Dishes

The Stress Free Diabetes Kitchen

Eggs and Egg Dishes

Asparagus Sformato

SERVES: 4 / SERVING SIZE: 1/4 RECIPE

This recipe was inspired by a dish I had in the town of Soave, Italy. You can use various sizes of soufflé or quiche dishes depending on whether you want to serve 2 or 4 people and whether you want to serve a light meal or first course. For a light meal or brunch, I used 2 8-ounce soufflé dishes. For a first course, I used 4 small ceramic quiche dishes.

» 1/4 pound asparagus spears
» 1 teaspoon extra virgin olive oil
» 1/4 cup minced shallot (about 1 large)
» Nonstick cooking spray
» 1 tablespoon bread crumbs
» 4 large eggs
» 1/2 cup 1% milk
» 1/2 teaspoon fine sea salt
» 1/4 teaspoon finely ground black pepper
» 2 tablespoons finely grated Parmigiano-Reggiano cheese
» 12 medium tomato slices

{ COOK'S TIP: }
For four servings, bake 15 minutes; for two servings, bake 23 minutes.

1. Preheat oven to 400°F.

2. Cut the tips off of the asparagus, just below the tip itself. Slice the remainder of the asparagus into 1/4-inch thick rounds. Sauté the asparagus and shallot in the olive oil for 2–3 minutes. Set aside to cool.

3. Spray baking dishes with nonstick cooking spray. Sprinkle each dish with some of the bread crumbs.

4. In a small bowl, whisk together the eggs, milk, salt, and pepper.

5. Divide the asparagus among the baking dishes. Pour some of the egg mixture into each dish. Top with cheese. Place on baking sheet. Bake 15–23 minutes, or until puffed and golden. Top each dish with three tomato slices.

Exchanges/Choices		
1/2 Carbohydrate	Calories 135	Potassium 365 mg
1 Med-Fat Meat	Calories from Fat 65	Total Carbohydrate 9 g
1/2 Fat	Total Fat 7.0 g	Dietary Fiber 2 g
	Saturated Fat 2.5 g	Sugars 4 g
	Trans Fat 0.0 g	Protein 10 g
	Cholesterol 190 mg	Phosphorus 185 mg
	Sodium 415 mg	

Scrambled Egg Tortilla with Avocado & Tomato

SERVES: 1 / SERVING SIZE: 1 TORTILLA

» 1 large egg
» Pinch fine sea salt
» 1/8 teaspoon ground black pepper
» 1 tablespoon shredded, fat-free cheddar cheese
» Nonstick cooking spray
» 1 whole-wheat tortilla (8-inch diameter)
» 1 plum tomato, chopped
» 1/4 Haas avocado, sliced
» 1 tablespoon chopped fresh cilantro or parsley

1. Scramble eggs in small bowl. Add salt, pepper, and cheese.

2. Lightly spray small sauté pan with nonstick cooking spray. Add scrambled egg mixture and cook to desired doneness.

3. Place eggs on one half of tortilla. Add tomato, avocado, and cilantro. Fold tortilla and serve.

{ COOK'S TIP:
Scramble eggs on medium for softer scrambled eggs. }

Exchanges/Choices		
2 Starch	Calories 290	Potassium 525 mg
1 Med-Fat Meat	Calories from Fat 100	Total Carbohydrate 35 g
1 Fat	Total Fat 11.0 g	Dietary Fiber 7 g
	Saturated Fat 2.5 g	Sugars 2 g
	Trans Fat 0.0 g	Protein 15 g
	Cholesterol 185 mg	Phosphorus 275 mg
	Sodium 555 mg	

Tomato Basil Frittata

SERVES: 6 / SERVING SIZE: 1/6 RECIPE

This frittata makes great use of leftover spaghetti. If you like spicy dishes, use crushed red pepper flakes instead of black pepper. Serve with a salad or fruit and you'll have a high-protein, quick, and easy meal. This can also be served at room temperature for a picnic or brown bag dish. Thank you Val and Laurie for Sharing!

» 6 large eggs
» 1/2 teaspoon fine sea salt
» 1/2 teaspoon ground black pepper, or crushed red pepper flakes
» 1 cup basil leaves, chopped
» 1/4 cup oregano leaves, chopped
» 1/3 cup grated Parmigiano-Reggiano cheese (additional for garnish, if desired)
» 3 cups sliced cherry or grape tomatoes
» 1/2 pound cooked spaghetti
» Nonstick cooking spray

1. Whisk eggs in large mixing bowl. Add salt, pepper, basil, oregano, and cheese. Mix well. Add tomatoes and spaghetti and mix well.

2. Brush sauté pan lightly with extra virgin olive oil. Add egg mixture. Cook on medium-high heat for about 7 minutes, or until the bottom is golden.

3. Place dinner plate on top of sauté pan. Turn the pan over so that the frittata is bottom side up on the plate. Slide frittata back into the sauté pan and cook until the second side is golden, about 4–5 minutes. You can cover the pan to cook more quickly, if desired.

4. Once done, sprinkle with additional grated cheese, if desired. Cover to melt cheese and keep warm. Cut into wedges and serve.

Exchanges/Choices		
1/2 Starch	Calories 165	Potassium 345 mg
1 Vegetable	Calories from Fat 55	Total Carbohydrate 16 g
1 Med-Fat Meat	Total Fat 6.0 g	Dietary Fiber 2 g
1/2 Fat	Saturated Fat 2.5 g	Sugars 3 g
	Trans Fat 0.0 g	Protein 11 g
	Cholesterol 190 mg	Phosphorus 175 mg
	Sodium 300 mg	

Sunshine Breakfast Pizza

SERVES: 1 / SERVING SIZE: 1 PIZZA

This bright, cheery breakfast pizza will start your day off right with the goodness of eggs, tomato, and mozzarella. The warmth of the egg enhances the flavor of the tomato and melts the cheese.

» Nonstick cooking spray
» 1 large egg
» Pinch fine sea salt
» Pinch freshly ground black pepper
» 1 sandwich/deli whole-wheat thin/flatbread
» 1 large plum tomato, sliced
» 1 1/2 tablespoons grated mozzarella cheese
» 2–3 basil leaves, chopped

1. Spray pan with nonstick cooking spray. Crack egg in sauté pan. Cook sunny side up and as the white becomes opaque, sprinkle with salt and pepper. Cover and cook to desired doneness.

2. Meanwhile, place toasted flatbread on serving plate. Top with slices of plum tomato and sprinkle with mozzarella and basil. Once egg is cooked, top the flatbread with egg.

Exchanges/Choices		
1 Vegetable	Calories 210	Potassium 395 mg
1 Med-Fat Meat	Calories from Fat 65	Total Carbohydrate 25 g
1/2 Fat	Total Fat 7.0 g	Dietary Fiber 6 g
	Saturated Fat 2.5 g	Sugars 5 g
	Trans Fat 0.0 g	Protein 14 g
	Cholesterol 190 mg	Phosphorus 250 mg
	Sodium 460 mg	

Open Face Egg & Spinach Salad Sandwich

SERVES: 1 / SERVING SIZE: 1 SANDWICH

This one dish meal is colorful, fresh, quick, easy, and delicious! Just right for one or more, especially after a trip to the Farmer's Market.

» 1 large egg, hard cooked
» 1/3 cup chopped tomato (about 1 small or 1/2 of a medium tomato)
» 1/2 cup corn kernels, lightly steamed, or use a leftover ear of fresh corn on the cob
» 1/4 cup sliced scallion, 1–2 scallions, depending on their size
» 1 tablespoon chopped flat Italian parsley
» 1 teaspoon extra virgin olive oil
» 1 teaspoon white balsamic vinegar
» 1/16 teaspoon fine sea salt
» 1/8 teaspoon freshly ground black pepper
» 1 slice (1 1/2-ounce) rustic whole-grain bread (such as ciabatta or round Italian sliced bread)
» 1 cup baby spinach

1. Place egg in a pan just large enough to hold it. Add enough cold water to cover egg by 1 inch. Bring to a boil. Once the water comes to a boil, watch carefully. Boil 30 seconds to 1 minute. Turn heat off and cover. (Let sit 18 minutes. Note: Boiling the egg too long results in a green ring around the yolk; however, it is still safe to eat.)

2. Mix together the tomato, corn, scallion, parsley, olive oil, vinegar, salt, and pepper. Set aside to let the flavors blend. This can be done ahead of time.

3. Toast the bread and place it on a large plate. Lay the spinach on top of the bread.

4. Slice the egg into 5–6 slices and lay them on top of the spinach. Spoon the tomato corn mixture onto the sandwich and serve.

Exchanges/Choices		
2 Starch	Calories 330	Potassium 870 mg
1 Vegetable	Calories from Fat 115	Total Carbohydrate 42 g
1 Med-Fat Meat	Total Fat 13.0 g	Dietary Fiber 8 g
1 Fat	Saturated Fat 2.8 g	Sugars 10 g
	Trans Fat 0.0 g	Protein 17 g
	Cholesterol 185 mg	Phosphorus 305 mg
	Sodium 455 mg	

Roasted Vegetable & Tomato Soufflé

SERVES: 4 / SERVING SIZE: 1/4 RECIPE

This recipe is a great do-ahead dish. You can prepare the soufflé up to one day before baking. You can also use this recipe for roasted vegetables to serve with other dishes or to tuck in an omelet.

Roasted Vegetables

» 1 medium zucchini (about 6-inches), quartered and sliced into 1/4-inch thick pieces
» 4 ounces cremini mushrooms, quartered
» 1 medium onion, roughly chopped
» 2 teaspoons extra virgin olive oil
» 1/4 teaspoon fine sea salt
» 1/4 teaspoon freshly ground black pepper

Soufflé

» 1 cup cherry or grape tomatoes, sliced in half
» 1/8 teaspoon salt
» 1/8 teaspoon pepper
» 7 large eggs
» 1 cup skim milk
» 1/4 cup minced fresh Italian parsley
» 1 teaspoon Dijon mustard
» Non-stick cooking spray
» 2 slices (1 1/2 ounce each) whole-grain rustic style bread, torn into bite-size pieces

1. Preheat oven to 400°F (convection if you have it). Line baking sheet with a sheet of parchment paper.

2. Place zucchini, mushrooms, and onion in large bowl. Add the olive oil, 1/2 teaspoon salt, and 1/4 teaspoon pepper. Toss well to coat the vegetables evenly. Place on baking sheet. Roast approximately 15 minutes, or until the edges begin to turn golden brown and vegetables are fork tender.

3. Place sliced tomatoes, 1/8 teaspoon salt, and 1/8 teaspoon pepper in the bowl with the other vegetables. Stir to mix well. Set aside.

4. Break eggs into large bowl. Add milk, parsley, and Dijon mustard. Whisk until ingredients are well combined.

(Continued on next page)

Exchanges/Choices		
1/2 Starch	Calories 260	Potassium 690 mg
2 Vegetable	Calories from Fat 110	Total Carbohydrate 21 g
2 Med-Fat Meat	Total Fat 12.0 g	Dietary Fiber 4 g
1/2 Fat	Saturated Fat 3.3 g	Sugars 9 g
	Trans Fat 0.0 g	Protein 18 g
	Cholesterol 325 mg	Phosphorus 355 mg
	Sodium 495 mg	

(Roasted Vegetable & Tomato Soufflé Continued)

5. Spray baking dish with nonstick spray. Place the bread in the bottom of the dish. Top with roasted veggies. Gently pour the egg mixture over all. Let sit 10 minutes, giving bread time to absorb the egg.

6. Bake in the center of the oven until golden and slightly puffed, approximately 20–25 minutes. Remove from oven. Let stand 5 minutes before cutting.

Individual Mushroom, Turkey & Egg Frittata

SERVES: 6 / SERVING SIZE: 1/6 RECIPE

» Nonstick cooking spray
» 3 links turkey breakfast sausage
» 3/4 cup chopped fresh mushrooms
» 1/3 cup chopped onion
» 4 large eggs
» 4 egg whites
» 1/3 cup skim milk
» 1/2 teaspoon fine sea salt
» 1/4 teaspoon freshly ground black pepper
» 1 1/2 teaspoons grated Parmigiano-Reggiano cheese

1. Preheat oven to 400°F.

2. Spray sauté pan with nonstick cooking spray. Remove casing from sausage links. Break sausage into small pieces and place in nonstick sauté pan. Add mushrooms and onions and sauté until sausage is cooked.

3. Line a muffin pan with foil liners. Divide the sausage mixture evenly among the muffin cups.

4. Place the eggs, egg whites, and milk in a bowl and whisk together. Add salt and pepper.

5. Pour egg mixture evenly into muffin cups. Top each serving with 1/4 teaspoon cheese.

6. Bake 30 minutes. Serve immediately.

Exchanges/Choices		
1 Med-Fat Meat	Calories 95	Potassium 175 mg
	Calories from Fat 40	Total Carbohydrate 2 g
	Total Fat 4.5 g	Dietary Fiber 0 g
	Saturated Fat 1.5 g	Sugars 1 g
	Trans Fat 0.0 g	Protein 10 g
	Cholesterol 135 mg	Phosphorus 120 mg
	Sodium 385 mg	

Savory Breakfast Casserole

SERVES: 4 / SERVING SIZE: 1/4 RECIPE

This dish is excellent for large groups when doubled or tripled and can be made ahead because it freezes beautifully. It makes a great brunch or light supper dish when served with a green or fruit salad.

» Nonstick cooking spray
» 2 large eggs
» 4 egg whites
» 1/4 teaspoon freshly ground pepper
» 1 cup skim milk
» 1/2 teaspoon Dijon mustard
» 1/4 pound (96% lean) ham slice, cut into 1/2-inch cubes, or 8 ounces cooked and crumbled breakfast sausage
» 2 thick slices (1 1/2 ounces each) good-quality bread, torn into 2-inch pieces
» 1/3 cup Cabot 50% reduced-fat shredded cheddar cheese

COOK'S TIP:
If you double this recipe, use a 9 × 13-inch pan. If you need to triple it, use an 8 × 8-inch pan and a 9 × 13-inch pan.

1. Spray casserole dish with nonstick cooking spray.

2. Place eggs and pepper in a large mixing bowl. Beat well. Add milk and mustard. Beat well.

3. Place ham or sausage and torn bread in bottom of casserole dish. Pour egg milk mixture over. Sprinkle with cheese. Cover and refrigerate 30 minutes or several hours. (You can also freeze uncooked in an aluminum foil pan. Do not defrost prior to cooking.)

4. Preheat oven to 350°F. Bake 20–25 minutes or until set. Casserole will be puffed in the center.

5. Cut into squares and serve hot. Leftovers reheat well in microwave.

Exchanges/Choices		
1 Carbohydrate	Calories 190	Potassium 310 mg
2 Lean Meat	Calories from Fat 55	Total Carbohydrate 16 g
1/2 Fat	Total Fat 6.0 g	Dietary Fiber 1 g
	Saturated Fat 2.2 g	Sugars 6 g
	Trans Fat 0.0 g	Protein 19 g
	Cholesterol 115 mg	Phosphorus 260 mg
	Sodium 665 mg	

Asparagus & Garden Herb Omelet

SERVES: 2 / SERVING SIZE: 1/2 OMELET

Spring is the time for asparagus and also a time when we begin to crave lighter foods. A recent writing assignment inspired me to incorporate asparagus with another wonderful food—the egg. Eggs are a great source of protein. They are also versatile and can be used in so many ways, anytime of the day.

» 4 large eggs
» Pinch of fine sea salt
» Pinch of freshly ground black pepper
» 1/4 cup of your favorite herbs (basil, chives, and Italian parsley)
» Nonstick cooking spray
» 4 spears of fresh asparagus, lightly sautéed or steamed
» 1/4 ounce shredded Gruyere cheese

1. Crack one whole egg and place in medium bowl. Separate three additional eggs and add the egg whites to the bowl with the whole egg. Add salt and pepper. Whisk until the eggs seem light and frothy. Add herbs. Whisk again until well blended.

2. Spray sauté pan with nonstick cooking spray. Heat pan to medium heat and add eggs. Cook slowly on medium until eggs begin to set. As the eggs set, lift the edge of the eggs, tilt pan, and allow the uncooked eggs from the top of the omelet to flow underneath the cooked eggs.

3. Once the egg mixture is almost all cooked, place asparagus on one half of the omelet. Sprinkle cheese over asparagus. Fold the other half over the asparagus. Let this cook until no liquid egg is present. Garnish with additional cheese and chopped herbs, if desired.

Exchanges/Choices
2 Lean Meat

Calories 95
   Calories from Fat 30
Total Fat 3.5 g
   Saturated Fat 1.5 g
   Trans Fat 0.0 g
Cholesterol 95 mg
Sodium 240 mg

Potassium 230 mg
Total Carbohydrate 2 g
   Dietary Fiber 1 g
   Sugars 1 g
Protein 12 g
Phosphorus 100 mg

Asparagus & Havarti Quiche

SERVES: 8 / SERVING SIZE: 1/8 RECIPE

You can make one 8-inch serving or 8 individual servings with this versatile no-crust recipe.

» Nonstick cooking spray
» 1 1/4 cups 2% evaporated milk
» 1/4 cup fat-free sour cream
» 1 teaspoon Dijon mustard
» 2 large eggs
» 4 large egg whites
» 3 tablespoons shredded Havarti cheese
» 1/4 cup chopped chives
» 1/2 pound fresh asparagus, steamed until fork tender
» Few grinds fresh black pepper
» Additional herbs for garnish

1. Preheat oven to 350°F. Place rack in center of oven. Spray baking dish with nonstick cooking spray.

2. Mix together milk, sour cream, mustard, eggs, and egg whites until well blended. Add cheese, chives, and asparagus. Blend well.

3. Pour mixture into baking dishes. Sprinkle with black pepper and additional herbs.

4. Bake until knife inserted in center comes out clean, approximately 35 minutes for one quiche and 20–25 for individual quiches. Let rest 10–15 minutes before serving. Leftovers can be eaten warm or cold.

Exchanges/Choices		
1/2 Carbohydrate	Calories 80	Potassium 220 mg
1 Lean Meat	Calories from Fat 25	Total Carbohydrate 7 g
	Total Fat 3.0 g	Dietary Fiber 0 g
	Saturated Fat 1.5 g	Sugars 5 g
	Trans Fat 0.0 g	Protein 7 g
	Cholesterol 55 mg	Phosphorus 135 mg
	Sodium 130 mg	

CHAPTER 6:
Vegetables

The Stress Free Diabetes Kitchen

Vegetables

Asparagus with Warm Shallot Vinaigrette & Orange Zest

SERVINGS: 6 / SERVING SIZE: 1/6 RECIPE

Warm Shallot Vinaigrette

» 3 tablespoons olive oil
» 2 tablespoons white wine vinegar
» 2 teaspoons honey
» 1 chopped shallot

» 2 pounds fresh asparagus
» 1 orange, zested

1. Heat olive oil in a small saucepan. Add white wine vinegar, honey, and shallot. Mix well and keep warm for drizzling over asparagus.

2. Hold the asparagus in one hand, and with the other hand, break off the opposite end. The stalk will break at the correct point. Discard bottom end.

3. Steam asparagus until fork tender. Timing will depend on the thickness of the stalks. Begin checking thin stalks at 4 minutes.

4. Lay asparagus on oval platter, drizzle with shallot vinaigrette, and garnish with orange zest. Serve at room temperature.

Exchanges/Choices	Calories 90	Potassium 190 mg
1 Vegetable	Calories from Fat 65	Total Carbohydrate 6 g
1 1/2 Fat	Total Fat 7.0 g	Dietary Fiber 2 g
	Saturated Fat 1.0 g	Sugars 3 g
	Trans Fat 0.0 g	Protein 2 g
	Cholesterol 0 mg	Phosphorus 45 mg
	Sodium 10 mg	

Asparagus with Hollandaise Sauce

SERVES: 6 / SERVING SIZE: 1/6 RECIPE

This Hollandaise is made with yogurt and no guilt!

» 2 pounds asparagus, washed and trimmed
» 12 tablespoons Hollandaise Sauce
» 2 tablespoons lemon juice
» 1 1/2 tablespoons melted butter
» 1 cup plain, nonfat yogurt
» 1/2 teaspoon fine sea salt
» 4 egg whites

1. Hold the asparagus in one hand, and with the other hand, break off the opposite end. The stalk will break at the correct point. Discard bottom end. Steam asparagus until fork tender. Timing will depend on the thickness of the stalks. Begin checking thin stalks at 4 minutes.

2. For hollandaise, whisk all remaining ingredients in a saucepan. Heat to medium and whisk until mixture barely begins to boil. Remove from heat.

3. Serve warm or chilled over asparagus.

COOK'S TIP:
When purchasing asparagus, look for dry tops and moist bottoms. The cut end should not be dry or woody looking. It should be standing in ice or a small pan of water in the produce department.

Exchanges/Choices		
1 Carbohydrate	Calories 70	Potassium 315 mg
1 Fat	Calories from Fat 20	Total Carbohydrate 7 g
	Total Fat 2.5 g	Dietary Fiber 2 g
	Saturated Fat 1.6 g	Sugars 5 g
	Trans Fat 0.1 g	Protein 6 g
	Cholesterol 5 mg	Phosphorus 125 mg
	Sodium 220 mg	

Roasted Asparagus with Breadcrumbs & Parmigiano

SERVES: 3 / SERVING SIZE: 1/3 RECIPE

This dish combines the complimentary flavors of Asparagus and Parmigiano-Reggiano. Purchase the real Parmigiano-Reggiano and you will get the most flavor from the least amount of cheese. Use a vegetable peeler to shave the Parmigiano and make sure the cheese is cold for best results.

» 1 pound asparagus (preferably thin)
» 1 large clove garlic, minced
» 1 teaspoon extra virgin olive oil
» 1/4 teaspoon fine sea salt
» 1/4 teaspoon freshly ground pepper
» 1 1/2 teaspoons good quality balsamic vinegar
» Fresh herb sprigs (for garnish)
» 1/4 cup bread crumbs
» 1/2 ounce freshly shaved Parmigiano-Reggiano

1. Preheat oven to 425°F. Line baking sheet with parchment.

2. Place trimmed asparagus and garlic in large bowl. Drizzle with olive oil, salt, and pepper. Toss gently. Place on baking sheet.

3. Roast to desired doneness, approximately 10 minutes for thin spears (cooking time will vary depending on the thickness of the asparagus).

4. Adjust seasonings to taste. Place on serving platter and sprinkle with balsamic vinegar. Garnish with fresh herbs and bread crumbs. Shave Parmigiano-Reggiano over all.

Exchanges/Choices		
1/2 Starch	Calories 85	Potassium 195 mg
1 Vegetable	Calories from Fat 30	Total Carbohydrate 10 g
1/2 Fat	Total Fat 3.5 g	Dietary Fiber 2 g
	Saturated Fat 1.4 g	Sugars 2 g
	Trans Fat 0.0 g	Protein 5 g
	Cholesterol 5 mg	Phosphorus 90 mg
	Sodium 305 mg	

Asparagus with Orange Glaze

SERVES: 6 / SERVING SIZE: 1/6 RECIPE

One way to jazz up a weeknight meal is by making a vegetable "extra special."

» 1 tablespoon minced fresh ginger (approximately 1 inch of fresh ginger)
» 2 pounds fresh asparagus
» 1/2 cup fresh orange juice
» Zest of 1 orange
» 2 teaspoons reduced-sodium soy sauce

1. Peel ginger and mince.

2. Hold the asparagus in one hand and with the other break off the opposite end. The stalk will break at the correct point. Discard bottom end.

3. Combine all of the ingredients, except the asparagus. Mix well with a wire whisk.

4. Place the asparagus in a shallow ovenproof dish. Cover with the sauce and refrigerate for at least 2 hours, turning occasionally, if possible.

5. Preheat the broiler. Broil the asparagus for 5–6 minutes or until tender, being careful not to overcook.

{ COOK'S TIP:
1-inch fresh ginger yields about 1 Tablespoon. }

Exchanges/Choices
1 Vegetable

Calories 30
  Calories from Fat 0
Total Fat 0.0 g
  Saturated Fat 0.0 g
  Trans Fat 0.0 g
Cholesterol 0 mg
Sodium 70 mg

Potassium 220 mg
Total Carbohydrate 6 g
  Dietary Fiber 2 g
  Sugars 3 g
Protein 2 g
Phosphorus 45 mg

Braised Baby Artichokes with Shallots

SERVES: 8 / SERVING SIZE: 1/8 RECIPE

When working with artichokes, you will want to prepare a bowl of acidulated water, which is simply water with a squeeze of fresh lemon. This prevents browning and keeps the artichokes looking fresh.

» 16 fresh baby artichokes
» 2 tablespoons extra virgin olive oil
» 2 garlic cloves, peeled and minced
» 4–6 shallots, thinly sliced
» 1/2–1 cup chicken or vegetable stock
» Fine sea salt
» Freshly ground pepper

1. Trim the stem end of the artichokes and remove outer leaves. Cut any prickly points off the artichokes. Place in acidulated water to keep from browning while trimming all the artichokes. Thinly slice the artichokes vertically (from stem end) into 1/4-inch thick slices.

2. Thinly film sauté pan with olive oil. Add garlic, shallots, and artichokes and cook 5–10 minutes over medium heat, until vegetables begin to soften. Add stock and cook until tender, approximately 10 more minutes. You can add additional stock to maintain a light sauce layer in the pan.

3. Season with salt and pepper to taste.

Exchanges/Choices		
2 Vegetable	Calories 70	Potassium 225 mg
1/2 Fat	Calories from Fat 30	Total Carbohydrate 9 g
	Total Fat 3.5 g	Dietary Fiber 6 g
	Saturated Fat 0.5 g	Sugars 1 g
	Trans Fat 0.0 g	Protein 2 g
	Cholesterol 0 mg	Phosphorus 55 mg
	Sodium 45 mg	

Braised Brussels Sprouts with Shallots & White Wine

SERVES: 6 / SERVING SIZE: 1/6 RECIPE

Brussels sprouts are a very underrated vegetable, mainly because most people over-cook them. This dish always gets rave reviews from my guests.

» 2 cups fresh Brussels sprouts
» 1 tablespoon extra virgin olive oil
» 2 garlic cloves, peeled and minced
» 1 cup thinly sliced shallots (about 4–6 shallots)
» 1/2–1 cup dry white wine, white vermouth, or chicken or vegetable stock
» 1/2 teaspoon fine sea salt
» Freshly ground pepper

1. Trim the stem end of the Brussels sprouts and remove outer leaves. Wash Brussels sprouts and thinly slice vertically (from stem end).

2. Heat extra virgin olive oil in sauté pan. Add garlic, shallots, and Brussels sprouts. Cook 3–5 minutes, until vegetables begin to soften. Add 1/2 cup wine or stock and cook until fork tender. Add additional wine or stock as necessary to keep pan moist. Season with salt and pepper to taste.

Exchanges/Choices		
1 Vegetable	Calories 50	Potassium 160 mg
1/2 Fat	Calories from Fat 20	Total Carbohydrate 5 g
	Total Fat 2.5 g	Dietary Fiber 1 g
	Saturated Fat 0.3 g	Sugars 1 g
	Trans Fat 0.0 g	Protein 1 g
	Cholesterol 0 mg	Phosphorus 30 mg
	Sodium 205 mg	

Grilled Vegetables

SERVES: 8 / SERVING SIZE: 1/8 RECIPE

This vegetable platter makes a lovely centerpiece for a buffet table. Consider your grill when slicing vegetables and cut them so that they will not fall through the grate. Varying the vegetable types and sizes will add to the appearance of your platter. Serve alongside just about any dish in the book.

» 1 large eggplant, unpeeled and sliced into 1/4-inch thick rounds
» 1/2 teaspoon fine sea salt
» 2 medium zucchini, unpeeled and sliced lengthwise into 1/4-inch thick rounds
» 2 sweet onions, peeled and sliced into very thin rounds
» 1 red bell pepper, cored and sliced into 1/4-inch thick rounds
» 1 green bell pepper, cored and sliced into 1/4-inch thick rounds
» 1 yellow bell pepper, cored and sliced into 1/4-inch thick rounds
» 2 tablespoons extra virgin olive oil
» 1/2 teaspoon freshly ground black pepper
» Fresh basil (for garnish)

1. Preheat grill or grill pan. Place eggplant in bowl large enough to hold all veggies. Lightly salt eggplant and let sit for 10 minutes.

2. Add remaining vegetables and toss with olive oil. Place on preheated grill and cook to desired doneness.

3. Season with salt and pepper as soon as vegetables are done. Garnish with fresh basil sprigs. This dish can be made early in the day and served at room temperature. Leftovers can be used for sandwiches or tossed with pasta.

{ COOK'S TIP:
Some vegetables only require grilling on one side. Heat kills vitamins and minerals, so the crispier the better. }

Exchanges/Choices		
3 Vegetable	Calories 105	Potassium 440 mg
1 Fat	Calories from Fat 35	Total Carbohydrate 18 g
	Total Fat 4.0 g	Dietary Fiber 4 g
	Saturated Fat 0.5 g	Sugars 9 g
	Trans Fat 0.0 g	Protein 2 g
	Cholesterol 0 mg	Phosphorus 65 mg
	Sodium 160 mg	

Roasted Vegetables

SERVINGS: 12 / SERVING SIZE: 1/2 CUP

Veggies are delicious when roasted. Their flavors are enhanced and the natural sugars are caramelized, which give them a nice crunch. Vary this recipe by using whatever veggies you like or roast one single vegetable at a time. I sometimes roast peeled beets or trimmed Brussels sprouts and even the naysayers always love them!

» 1 small eggplant, unpeeled, cut into 1-inch chunks
» 1/2 teaspoon fine sea salt
» 1 zucchini, sliced into 1-inch pieces
» 1 yellow squash, sliced into 1-inch pieces
» 10 ounces cremini mushrooms
» 4 shallots, peeled and quartered
» 1 red bell pepper, cut into 1-inch chunks
» 1 green bell pepper, cut into 1-inch chunks
» 1 yellow bell pepper, cut into 1-inch chunks
» 1 head garlic, cloves separated and peeled
» 2 tablespoons extra virgin olive oil
» Freshly ground pepper
» 2 tablespoons good quality balsamic vinegar
» Fresh herb sprigs (for garnish)

1. Preheat oven to 425°F.

2. Place eggplant in a large bowl. Lightly salt eggplant and let sit for 10 minutes. (This will prevent it from absorbing too much oil.) Add remaining vegetables and toss with olive oil.

3. Line baking sheet with parchment. Place vegetables on baking sheet. Sprinkle with salt and pepper to taste. Roast to desired doneness, approximately 20–30 minutes. Adjust seasonings to taste.

4. Place on serving platter and sprinkle with balsamic vinegar. Garnish with fresh herbs.

{ COOK'S TIP:
Toss with whole-grain pasta and serve at room temperature with a dressing of extra virgin olive oil and balsamic vinegar. }

Exchanges/Choices
2 Vegetable
1/2 Fat

Calories 65
    Calories from Fat 20
Total Fat 2.5 g
    Saturated Fat 0.4 g
    Trans Fat 0.0 g
Cholesterol 0 mg
Sodium 105 mg

Potassium 345 mg
Total Carbohydrate 10 g
    Dietary Fiber 2 g
    Sugars 4 g
Protein 2 g
Phosphorus 65 mg

Roasted Root Vegetables with Garlic

SERVES: 8 / SERVING SIZE: 1/8 RECIPE

This is a great way to incorporate less common veggies, such as parsnips and turnips into our diet. Roasting makes any veggie taste great!

» 3–4 turnips, scrubbed or peeled, cut into 1-inch chunks
» 3–4 carrots, scrubbed or peeled, cut into 1-inch chunks
3» –4 Yukon Gold potatoes, scrubbed, unpeeled, cut into 1-inch chunks
» 3–4 parsnips, scrubbed, peeled, cut into 1-inch chunks
» 8–12 shallots, peeled
» 1 head garlic, cloves separated and peeled
» 2 tablespoons extra virgin olive oil
» 1 teaspoon fine sea salt
» 1 teaspoon freshly ground pepper
» 1 Tablespoon balsamic vinegar
» Fresh herb sprigs (for garnish)

1. Preheat oven to 425°F.

2. Place all veggies in large bowl and toss with olive oil, salt, and pepper. Line baking sheet with parchment. Place vegetables on baking sheet.

3. Roast to desired doneness, approximately 40–45 minutes. Adjust seasonings to taste.

4. Place on serving platter and sprinkle with balsamic vinegar. Garnish with fresh herbs.

Exchanges/Choices	Calories 140	Potassium 540 mg
1 Starch	Calories from Fat 30	Total Carbohydrate 26 g
2 Vegetable	Total Fat 3.5 g	Dietary Fiber 5 g
1/2 Fat	Saturated Fat 0.5 g	Sugars 5 g
	Trans Fat 0.0 g	Protein 3 g
	Cholesterol 0 mg	Phosphorus 85 mg
	Sodium 330 mg	

Roasted Vegetable Strudel with Pesto

SERVES: 5 / SERVING SIZE: 1/5 RECIPE

This dish is beautiful. When made in individual servings, it is a great picnic or brown bag item.

» 5 sheets phyllo pastry (14 × 18-inch sheets)
» 2 cups Roasted Vegetables (page 104)
» 1/4 cup Parmigiano-Reggiano cheese, grated
» Olive oil spray

1. Thaw phyllo dough overnight in refrigerator, or for 3 hours at room temperature.

2. Preheat oven to 400°F. Sprinkle vegetables with Parmigiano-Reggiano. (For brown bagging, use half sheets of phyllo and make individual strudels.)

3. Lay phyllo on your work surface and cover with a damp towel. Take one sheet of phyllo and lay it on top of a baking sheet. Spray or brush with olive oil. Repeat this process with the remaining phyllo.

4. Spread vegetables over dough, leaving a 2-inch edge all the way around. Fold in short sides and begin rolling like a jellyroll. Place seam side down on baking sheet. Spray or brush lightly with olive oil.

5. Bake for 30 minutes or until golden brown and beautiful. Can be served warm or at room temperature. Drizzle with No Oil Pesto (page 107).

Exchanges/Choices		
1 Starch	Calories 145	Potassium 295 mg
2 Vegetable	Calories from Fat 40	Total Carbohydrate 23 g
1/2 Fat	Total Fat 4.5 g	Dietary Fiber 2 g
	Saturated Fat 1.2 g	Sugars 3 g
	Trans Fat 0.0 g	Protein 4 g
	Cholesterol 5 mg	Phosphorus 95 mg
	Sodium 200 mg	

No Oil Pesto

SERVES: 12 / SERVING SIZE: 1 TABLESPOON

This pesto is great when drizzled over Roasted Vegetable Strudel (page 106).

» 1 bunch fresh basil leaves
» 1 garlic clove
» 1/4 cup grated Parmigiano-Reggiano
   cheese
» 1/4 cup pignoli nuts (pine nuts)
» 1/4–1/2 cup vegetable stock

1. Place all ingredients in food processor and blend until smooth.

2. Drizzle over vegetable strudel.

Exchanges/Choices	Calories 25	Potassium 35 mg
1/2 Fat	Calories from Fat 20	Total Carbohydrate 1 g
	Total Fat 2.5 g	Dietary Fiber 0 g
	Saturated Fat 0.4 g	Sugars 0 g
	Trans Fat 0.0 g	Protein 1 g
	Cholesterol 0 mg	Phosphorus 30 mg
	Sodium 25 mg	

Veggie Stir Fry

SERVES: 2 / SERVING SIZE: 1/2 RECIPE

You can follow the stir-fry guidelines below and create any kind of stir-fry that you want, from Shrimp & Broccoli, to Beef & Green Beans. Experimenting with different types of veggies is a great way to get more veggies into your meal plan. A wok is not necessary, any large sauté pan will do. (See Stir-Fry Guidelines, page 8.)

» 1 tablespoon cornstarch
» 1 cup low-sodium vegetable broth
» 1 teaspoon light soy sauce
» 2 tablespoons peanut oil
» 2 large cloves garlic, peeled and sliced thinly
» 1-inch piece ginger, peeled and sliced thinly
» 2 cups fresh veggies of your choice, thinly sliced or cut into bite-size pieces (depending on the veggie)

1. Mix cornstarch, stock, and soy sauce. Set aside.

2. Heat oil in a large sauté pan, or wok. Add garlic and ginger and cook until golden. Remove.

3. Add veggies and cook until crisp tender. Add cornstarch mixture to pan. Cook until sauce is thickened and clear. Serve over brown rice.

Exchanges/Choices
2 Vegetable
3 Fat

Calories 175
   Calories from Fat 125
Total Fat 14.0 g
   Saturated Fat 2.3 g
   Trans Fat 0.0 g
Cholesterol 0 mg
Sodium 170 mg

Potassium 220 mg
Total Carbohydrate 12 g
   Dietary Fiber 2 g
   Sugars 4 g
Protein 2 g
Phosphorus 60 mg

Spring Peas with Fresh Mint

SERVES: 6 / SERVING SIZE: 1/6 RECIPE

This dish is traditionally made with fresh peas; however, if your life is too hectic, you can use a 16-ounce bag of frozen petite peas.

» 3 pounds fresh peas
» 1 tablespoon unsalted butter
» 1 cup fresh mint leaves
» 1/2 teaspoon fine sea salt
» 1/4 teaspoon freshly ground black pepper

1. Shell peas. Steam them for 3–5 minutes. Drain.

2. Melt butter in sauté pan. Add mint and mix well. Add peas and heat thoroughly. Season with salt and pepper.

Exchanges/Choices		
1 Starch	Calories 85	Potassium 260 mg
1/2 Fat	Calories from Fat 20	Total Carbohydrate 13 g
	Total Fat 2.0 g	Dietary Fiber 5 g
	Saturated Fat 1.3 g	Sugars 5 g
	Trans Fat 0.1 g	Protein 5 g
	Cholesterol 5 mg	Phosphorus 95 mg
	Sodium 200 mg	

Oven-Baked Eggplant Parmigiano

SERVES: 8 / SERVING SIZE: 1/8 RECIPE

Marinara Sauce

» 1 tablespoon extra virgin olive oil
» 2 cloves garlic, chopped
» 1 28-ounce can tomato purée or crushed tomatoes
» 1 cup fresh basil leaves

Eggplant

» 1/2 teaspoon salt
» 1 large eggplant, sliced into 1/2-inch thick pieces
» 3 large eggs
» 1 cup Italian-style bread crumbs
» 1/4 cup grated Parmigiano-Reggiano cheese
» 1/2 teaspoon black pepper

1. Preheat oven to 400°F. Place the olive oil in the bottom of a large saucepan. Add garlic and cook until fragrant, but don't let it get dark brown. Add tomatoes and basil. Bring to a low boil, reduce heat, and simmer.

2. Lightly salt the eggplant. (This will prevent eggplant from absorbing too much olive oil.)

3. Crack eggs and scramble with a fork in large dish or pie plate.

4. Place breadcrumbs, cheese, and pepper in large dish or pie plate. Mix well.

5. Dip eggplant in eggs, then dip in bread crumb mixture. Place eggplant on parchment-lined baking sheet and bake, about 20 minutes or until eggplant is golden brown.

6. Top with a spoon of marinara sauce and cheese, if desired. Return to oven for 2–3 minutes to melt cheese. Serve.

Exchanges/Choices		
1/2 Starch	Calories 150	Potassium 615 mg
3 Vegetable	Calories from Fat 40	Total Carbohydrate 24 g
1 Fat	Total Fat 4.5 g	Dietary Fiber 5 g
	Saturated Fat 1.2 g	Sugars 8 g
	Trans Fat 0.0 g	Protein 6 g
	Cholesterol 55 mg	Phosphorus 110 m
	Sodium 385 mg	

Sweet Potato and Orange Casserole

SERVES: 8 / SERVING SIZE: 1/8 RECIPE

» 2 pounds sweet potatoes, cut in half
» 3 navel oranges, peeled and cut into 1/4-inch slices
» 2 teaspoons orange zest
» 1 tablespoons cornstarch
» 1 cup orange juice
» 3 tablespoons honey or maple syrup
» 1/8 teaspoon ground cloves
» 2 tablespoons slivered almonds

1. Place potatoes in saucepan and cover with water. Boil until fork tender. Drain, cool, peel, and cut sweet potatoes into 1/4-inch slices. Mix gently with orange slices. Transfer to a 9 × 13-inch baking dish.

2. In a 1-quart saucepan, mix orange zest, and cornstarch with juice, honey, and cloves. Cook over medium heat, stirring constantly until thickened. Pour over sweet potatoes. Top with slivered almonds.

Exchanges/Choices	Calories 155	Potassium 400 mg
1 Starch	Calories from Fat 15	Total Carbohydrate 35 g
1 1/2 Fruit	Total Fat 1.5 g	Dietary Fiber 4 g
	Saturated Fat 0.1 g	Sugars 19 g
	Trans Fat 0.0 g	Protein 2 g
	Cholesterol 0 mg	Phosphorus 60 mg
	Sodium 30 mg	

Mashed Celery Root with Garlic

SERVES: 4 / SERVING SIZE: 1/4 RECIPE

I have seen people pick up a celery root in the produce aisle and not know what it is. I wish grocers put up more signs and explanations! This ugly, brown, knob has great fresh flavor and is a great substitute for higher starch side dishes. It is also wonderful used as a substitute for mashed potatoes.

» 2 pounds celery root or celeriac, cut into quarters or eighths and peeled
» 2 cloves garlic
» 1/2 teaspoon fine sea salt
» 1/4 teaspoon freshly ground black pepper
» 1/2 cup skim milk
» 1/4 cup chopped flat Italian parsley

1. Place celery root, garlic, salt, and pepper in a 4-quart saucepan and cover with water. Bring to a boil and cook until tender, about 15 minutes (similar to mashed potatoes).

2. Drain and mash with a large fork or potato masher. Stir in milk and parsley.

{ COOK'S TIP:
Place in small ramekins and heat in the oven at serving time. Serve instead of potatoes, rice, or pasta. }

Exchanges/Choices		
1 Starch	Calories 65	Potassium 400 mg
	Calories from Fat 0	Total Carbohydrate 14 g
	Total Fat 0.0 g	Dietary Fiber 2 g
	Saturated Fat 0.0 g	Sugars 4 g
	Trans Fat 0.0 g	Protein 3 g
	Cholesterol 0 mg	Phosphorus 165 mg
	Sodium 430 mg	

Spaghetti Squash with Light Marinara Sauce

SERVES: 6 / SERVING SIZE: 1/6 RECIPE

This is a fun dish to serve kids—they get a real kick out of the name.

Spaghetti Squash

» 1 medium spaghetti squash (about 2 pounds), washed
» 1 tablespoon extra virgin olive oil
» 1 tablespoon finely grated Parmigiano-Reggiano

Marinara

» 14 plum tomatoes, chopped
» 2 cloves garlic, chopped
» 1 shallot, minced
» 1 tablespoon extra virgin olive oil
» Freshly ground pepper
» 1/2 teaspoon fine sea salt
» 1 cup fresh basil leaves
» 6 teaspoon Parmigiano-Reggiano (optional)

1. Pierce spaghetti squash with a fork in several places and place in microwave on high until skin is soft, approximately 10–15 minutes. Let cool.

2. While squash is cooking, combine all marinara ingredients in a medium-sized bowl.

3. Tear basil leaves and add to tomato mixture. Sauté lightly until tomatoes are softened.

4. Cut squash in half and make "spaghetti." Using a fork, pull out individual strands of "spaghetti." Toss spaghetti squash with olive oil and Parmigiano-Reggiano.

5. Place squash in a pie plate. Top with light marinara and a sprinkling of Parmigiano-Reggiano.

6. Toss with cooked pasta or serve over spaghetti squash.

Exchanges/Choices	Calories 95	Potassium 485 mg
2 Vegetable	Calories from Fat 45	Total Carbohydrate 12 g
1 Fat	Total Fat 5.0 g	Dietary Fiber 3 g
	Saturated Fat 0.9 g	Sugars 6 g
	Trans Fat 0.0 g	Protein 2 g
	Cholesterol 0 mg	Phosphorus 60 mg
	Sodium 225 mg	

Grilled Eggplant with Spinach Pesto Stuffing

SERVES: 4 / SERVING SIZE: 1/4 RECIPE

This is a great do-ahead dish. The individual serving size makes it lovely on the plate.

Spinach Pesto

» 4 cups fresh baby spinach
» 1-cup fresh parsley
» 1/2 cup grated Parmigiano-Reggiano,
    plus extra for garnish
» 6 cloves garlic
» 1/2 cup low-sodium vegetable stock

» 2 small eggplants
» 1 teaspoon olive oil

1. Place spinach, parsley, cheese, and garlic in a food processor and process until smooth. Add stock until you reach desired consistency.

2. Cut eggplants in half lengthwise. Brush with olive oil and grill until flesh is soft. You can also bake these in the oven at 400°F for 20–30 minutes.

3. Spread spinach pesto on top of eggplant and garnish with a light sprinkling of Parmigiano-Reggiano. Place under broiler to warm and brown cheese.

Exchanges/Choices		
3 Vegetable	Calories 160	Potassium 640 mg
1 1/2 Fat	Calories from Fat 70	Total Carbohydrate 20 g
	Total Fat 8.0 g	Dietary Fiber 6 g
	Saturated Fat 2.2 g	Sugars 6 g
	Trans Fat 0.0 g	Protein 7 g
	Cholesterol 5 mg	Phosphorus 135 mg
	Sodium 220 mg	

Peanut Sauced Veggie Angel Hair

Serves: 4 / Serving Size: 1/4 recipe

If you can get hold of a "julienne peeler" your veggies will definitely look like angel hair.

» 1 tablespoon canola oil
» 1 medium onion, diced
» 2 carrots, julienne
» 2 stalks celery, julienne
» 1 8-ounce can diced water chestnuts
» 2 cups low-sodium broth
» 1 tablespoon natural peanut butter

1. Add oil and onion to a saucepan and heat over medium heat. Cook for 2–3 minutes, until onion begins to become translucent. Add carrots, celery, water chestnuts, some broth, and peanut butter.

2. Toss and cook until carrots and celery are tender. Add more broth to achieve sauce-like consistency. Serve.

Exchanges/Choices	Calories 120	Potassium 355 mg
3 Vegetable	Calories from Fat 55	Total Carbohydrate 14 g
1 Fat	Total Fat 6.0 g	Dietary Fiber 4 g
	Saturated Fat 0.6 g	Sugars 5 g
	Trans Fat 0.0 g	Protein 2 g
	Cholesterol 0 mg	Phosphorus 70 mg
	Sodium 135 mg	

Sautéed Spinach

SERVES: 1 / SERVING SIZE: 1 RECIPE

This is the quickest and most convenient veggie side dish I have ever made. You can use this with anything and also season it with anything you like, from lemon juice to balsamic vinegar to garlic powder and extra virgin olive oil.

» 1 6-ounce bag baby spinach

1. Rinse spinach in a colander and place in a large sauté pan. Cook with only the water that clings to the leaves. Cover and cook about 3 minutes.

Exchanges/Choices	Calories 40	Potassium 950 mg
1 Vegetable	Calories from Fat 5	Total Carbohydrate 6 g
	Total Fat 0.5 g	Dietary Fiber 4 g
	Saturated Fat 0.1 g	Sugars 1 g
	Trans Fat 0.0 g	Protein 5 g
	Cholesterol 0 mg	Phosphorus 85 mg
	Sodium 135 mg	

Spinaci Alla Fiorentina

SERVES: 8 / SERVING SIZE: 1/8 RECIPE

This dish is reminiscent of one that I prepared in cooking school in Tuscany.

» 1 cup pignoli nuts (pine nuts), toasted
» 2 10-ounce bags baby spinach, washed and drained
» 3 cloves garlic, finely minced
» Salt to taste
» Pepper to taste
» 1/2 cup raisins

1. Place pignoli nuts in dry sauté pan and heat. Watch closely until nuts begin to turn golden brown. Remove from pan so that they do not over-cook. Cool. (You can also store these in an airtight container in the refrigerator for future use.)

2. Place spinach and garlic in large sauté pan. Cook with the water that clings to spinach. Season with salt and pepper. Add Pignoli and raisins. Cook until dish is hot and well blended.

3. Garnish with a drizzle of extra virgin olive oil and vinegar, if desired.

Exchanges/Choices		
1/2 Fruit	Calories 160	Potassium 570 mg
1 Vegetable	Calories from Fat 110	Total Carbohydrate 12 g
2 1/2 Fat	Total Fat 12.0 g	Dietary Fiber 3 g
	Saturated Fat 0.9 g	Sugars 6 g
	Trans Fat 0.0 g	Protein 5 g
	Cholesterol 0 mg	Phosphorus 145 mg
	Sodium 55 mg	

Grilled Escarole with Toasted Garlic, Beans, and Lemon Thyme Vinaigrette

SERVES: 4 / SERVING SIZE: 1/4 RECIPE

This beautiful salad can be made ahead of time and kept at room temperature until serving time. The toasted garlic is a tasty treat and great on other dishes as well. The beans make this a very satisfying dish packed with protein.

» 1 head escarole, cut lengthwise in quarters through core (so the leaves stay intact), washed and dried
» 1/4 cup olive oil, plus extra for brushing on greens
» 8 large cloves garlic, sliced lengthwise
» 1 lemon, juiced
» 8 sprigs fresh thyme
» 1 15-ounce can small white beans, drained and rinsed well
» 1/2 teaspoon fine sea salt
» 1/2 teaspoon freshly ground black pepper
» Lemon slices (for garnish)

1. Lightly brush escarole with olive oil. Grill or sauté until cut sides are lightly browned and only slightly wilted. Place on platter or individual salad plates and hold at room temperature.

2. Place 1/4 cup olive oil in small saucepan. Heat and then add sliced garlic. Watch carefully and cook until golden. Remove garlic from oil with slotted spoon.

3. Mix the warm olive oil with lemon juice, thyme, and beans. Add salt and pepper to taste. Set aside. (This step can be done several hours ahead of time.)

4. Place 1 piece of escarole on each plate. Divide beans and dressing among the four plates and sprinkle with toasted garlic. Garnish with lemon slice and serve at room temperature.

{ **COOK'S TIP:**
To wash escarole: fill your sink with water and swish the lettuce around to release dirt. }

Exchanges/Choices		
1 Starch	Calories 250	Potassium 545 mg
1 Vegetable	Calories from Fat 145	Total Carbohydrate 22 g
3 Fat	Total Fat 16.0 g	Dietary Fiber 9 g
	Saturated Fat 2.3 g	Sugars 1 g
	Trans Fat 0.0 g	Protein 7 g
	Cholesterol 0 mg	Phosphorus 125 mg
	Sodium 445 mg	

Oven Roasted Potatoes with Rosemary & Garlic

SERVES: 6 / SERVING SIZE: 1/6 RECIPE

I think that this is my absolute favorite way to serve potatoes!

» 2 tablespoons fresh rosemary
» 3 pounds potatoes, such as Yukon Gold or Red Bliss
» 8 garlic cloves, whole, peeled
» 1 tablespoon extra virgin olive oil
» 1 teaspoon fine sea salt
» 1/2 teaspoon freshly ground pepper or more, if desired

1. Preheat oven to 425°F. Strip rosemary from stems. Slightly bruise with chef's knife.

2. Place potatoes, rosemary, and garlic in large mixing bowl. Toss with olive oil, salt, and pepper.

3. Place mixture on a parchment-lined baking sheet in a single layer.

4. Roast in oven 30 minutes to 1 hour (depending on size of potato), or until fork tender and golden brown.

Exchanges/Choices	Calories 185	Potassium 895 mg
2 1/2 Starch	Calories from Fat 20	Total Carbohydrate 38 g
	Total Fat 2.5 g	Dietary Fiber 5 g
	Saturated Fat 0.4 g	Sugars 2 g
	Trans Fat 0.0 g	Protein 4 g
	Cholesterol 0 mg	Phosphorus 125 mg
	Sodium 405 mg	

Purple Potato Salad with Green Beans and Tear Drop Tomatoes

SERVES: 8 / SERVING SIZE: 1/8 RECIPE

I love cooking with lots of beautiful colors. It's like taking a Nutrition 101 course without having to crack a book—the more colors you have, the more different nutrients you have on your plate.

» 3 pounds purple potatoes (or your favorite potato, if purple are not available)
» 1 pound green beans, stemmed
» 1/4 cup red wine vinegar
» 1 teaspoon Dijon mustard
» Fine sea salt
» Freshly ground pepper
» 1/4 cup extra virgin olive oil
» 1 pint red teardrop, cherry, or grape tomatoes, washed and dried
» 1/2 cup fresh basil, torn at last minute

1. Cut potatoes into bite-size pieces and boil until tender. Drain well.

2. Steam green beans for 6–8 minutes in a steamer pot or regular pot.

3. Place vinegar, mustard, salt, and pepper into a small bowl. Slowly whisk in olive oil until combined well.

4. Place potatoes and green beans in a large bowl and toss with dressing. Add tomatoes and basil.

5. Serve at room temperature.

Exchanges/Choices		
2 1/2 Starch	Calories 255	Potassium 900 mg
1 Vegetable	Calories from Fat 65	Total Carbohydrate 45 g
1 Fat	Total Fat 7.0 g	Dietary Fiber 6 g
	Saturated Fat 1.0 g	Sugars 4 g
	Trans Fat 0.0 g	Protein 5 g
	Cholesterol 0 mg	Phosphorus 195 mg
	Sodium 15 mg	

Roasted Tomato with Basil, Speck & Asiago

SERVES: 3 / SERVING SIZE: 1/3 RECIPE

I enjoyed an oven-roasted tomato similar to this when visiting friends in Verona, Italy. Since then, this has become a side dish staple in my kitchen for both weeknight and company dinners. It is especially nice because the Speck and Asiago turn even winter tomatoes into something special.

» 2 large or 3 medium-size tomatoes
» 1 ounce finely diced Speck
» 1/2 ounce shredded Asiago-Staggionato
» 2 tablespoons fresh bread crumbs
» 1/4 cup minced fresh basil leaves

1. Preheat oven to 450°F.

2. Cut tomatoes in half horizontally. Place on parchment-lined baking sheet and roast until they begin to soften, about 10 minutes.

3. Mix remaining ingredients together and mound on top of the tomato halves. Return to oven and roast another 8–10 minutes until topping is crispy.

Exchanges/Choices	Calories 75	Potassium 420 mg
1 Vegetable	Calories from Fat 25	Total Carbohydrate 7 g
1 Lean Meat	Total Fat 3.0 g	Dietary Fiber 2 g
	Saturated Fat 1.4 g	Sugars 4 g
	Trans Fat 0.0 g	Protein 6 g
	Cholesterol 10 mg	Phosphorus 95 mg
	Sodium 230 mg	

Sautéed Kale with Extra Virgin Olive Oil, Garlic & Crushed Red Pepper

SERVES: 3 / SERVING SIZE: 1/3 RECIPE

Kale is a powerhouse of nutrients. Some stores carry it in bags already washed and cut, but remember that some of the nutritional value is lost when you purchase cut veggies.

» 2 tablespoons extra virgin olive oil
» 3–4 cloves garlic, minced
» Crushed red pepper, to taste
» 1 large bunch kale, washed, dried, and cut into bite-size pieces

1. Place extra virgin olive oil in sauté pan. Add garlic and crushed red pepper and heat until garlic become fragrant. Add Kale and sauté until wilted, adding more extra virgin olive oil, if desired.

Exchanges/Choices		
2 Vegetable	Calories 130	Potassium 425 mg
2 Fat	Calories from Fat 90	Total Carbohydrate 10 g
	Total Fat 10.0 g	Dietary Fiber 2 g
	Saturated Fat 1.3 g	Sugars 7 g
	Trans Fat 0.0 g	Protein 3 g
	Cholesterol 0 mg	Phosphorus 55 mg
	Sodium 40 mg	

Garlic Mashed Potatoes

SERVES: 8 / SERVING SIZE: 1/8 RECIPE

These mashed potatoes are heart healthy and delicious. You get great flavor without cream or butter and you add back all the nutrients by using the cooking liquid instead of milk.

» 12 Yukon Gold potatoes, peeled and cut into 1-inch cubes
» 6 cloves garlic, peeled
» 1 teaspoon fine sea salt
» 4–6 cups low-sodium chicken, vegetable, or beef stock
» Freshly ground pepper to taste

1. Place potatoes, garlic, and salt in heavy saucepan. Add stock and additional water to cover. Boil until potatoes are fork tender, about 10 minutes.

2. Drain liquid from potatoes and reserve in a bowl to add back to potatoes.

3. Place potatoes in mixer bowl. Mix until smooth and add the hot cooking liquid until potatoes are desired consistency. Add black pepper to taste.

COOK'S TIP:
» Leftover cooking liquid can be used in sauces or soups.
» These potatoes can be frozen in an oven-proof casserole dish, defrosted, and reheated in a 350°F, approximately 45 minutes.

Exchanges/Choices	Calories 105	Potassium 470 mg
1 1/2 Starch	Calories from Fat 0	Total Carbohydrate 23 g
	Total Fat 0.0 g	Dietary Fiber 2 g
	Saturated Fat 0.1 g	Sugars 1 g
	Trans Fat 0.0 g	Protein 3 g
	Cholesterol 0 mg	Phosphorus 65 mg
	Sodium 345 mg	

CHAPTER 7:
Rice, Grain, Pasta & Sauces

The Stress Free Diabetes Kitchen

Rice, Grain, Pasta & Sauces

Farmer's Market Pasta

SERVES: 8 / SERVING SIZE: 1/8 RECIPE

When I make a trip to the Farmer's Market, I never know what I am going to find. I love having my recipes defined by the seasonal vegetables available. This dish is so versatile, because you can substitute any vegetable, depending on what's in season.

» 1 pound whole-wheat pasta of your choice, cooked al dente
» 2 garlic cloves, minced
» 2 tablespoons extra virgin olive oil
» 4 cups veggies of your choice, sliced or diced
» Fine sea salt
» Freshly ground black pepper
» Parmigiano-Reggiano (optional)

1. Cook pasta according to package directions.

2. Place garlic and olive oil in large sauté pan. Add veggies and sauté to desired doneness. Season with salt and pepper. Toss with pasta.

3. Garnish with grated Parmigiano-Reggiano, if desired.

Exchanges/Choices
2 1/2 Starch
1 Vegetable
1/2 Fat

Calories 260
　Calories from Fat 40
Total Fat 4.5 g
　Saturated Fat 0.6 g
　Trans Fat 0.0 g
Cholesterol 0 mg
Sodium 15 mg

Potassium 170 mg
Total Carbohydrate 48 g
　Dietary Fiber 7 g
　Sugars 4 g
Protein 8 g
Phosphorus 125 mg

Val's Long Bean Pasta

SERVES: 8 / SERVING SIZE: 1/8 RECIPE

This delicious and healthy recipe was served to me by a close friend who also graciously shared it for this cookbook. His mother used to prepare this dish in Italy using a thin, delicate green bean that we don't find in America. He found that Asian Long Beans come close to the beans used by his mama.

» 2 pounds Asian long beans, stem end trimmed and cut into 6-inch lengths,
» 28 ounces whole San Marzano tomatoes
» 4 tablespoons extra virgin olive oil
» Pinch of crushed red pepper
» 1 medium onion, chopped fine
» 2 tablespoons chopped fresh garlic
» 1 teaspoon sea or kosher salt
» Freshly ground black pepper to taste
» 1 pound pasta (preferably long pasta, such as Perciatelli or Fettuccine), cooked al dente
» Generous handful of hand-torn fresh basil
» 4 tablespoons grated Pecorino Romano or Parmigiano-Reggiano cheese

1. In a large pot, bring a generous amount of unsalted water to boil. Boil the beans until they have lost their crispness, but are still somewhat firm and not cooked fully through (Note: the beans will cook in the sauce for another 10 to 20 minutes, so you don't want to boil them until they are totally tender.) Once beans are done, drain and rinse in cold water to stop any further cooking. Set beans aside.

2. Heat the olive oil and crushed red pepper in a large saucepan over medium-high heat. Add onion and sauté until the onion becomes slightly translucent. Add garlic and cook until fragrant, about 30 seconds

(Continued on next page)

Exchanges/Choices		
3 Starch	Calories 375	Potassium 555 mg
3 Vegetable	Calories from Fat 80	Total Carbohydrate 61 g
1 1/2 Fat	Total Fat 9.0 g	Dietary Fiber 8 g
	Saturated Fat 1.8 g	Sugars 6 g
	Trans Fat 0.0 g	Protein 13 g
	Cholesterol 0 mg	Phosphorus 190 mg
	Sodium 460 mg	

(Val's Long Bean Pasta Continued)

3. Crush the tomatoes in a bowl. Turn heat to medium-high and add the tomatoes. Bring to boil and immediately reduce to simmer.

4. Stir in salt and freshly ground black pepper to taste. Simmer tomato sauce for at least 20 minutes

5. Add the beans and simmer for another 10 to 20 minutes until the beans are tender but firm. (Do not overcook the beans. They should still be somewhat firm when done.)

6. In a large pot of salted boiling water, cook pasta to al dente. Reserve 1/2 cup cooking liquid and drain the pasta. Add basil, grated cheese, and pasta to the sauce. If sauce is dry, add some of the reserved pasta water. Serve immediately.

{ COOK'S TIP:
» The sauce can be prepared ahead and refrigerated for up to one week or frozen.
» Asian long beans may be difficult to find if you do not have an Asian market available (See variation idea on page 8.) }

Quick Fresh Herb Marinara Sauce for Pizza, Pasta, or Meatballs

SERVES: 4 / SERVING SIZE: 1/2 CUP

» 2 tablespoons extra virgin olive oil
» 4 cloves garlic, minced
» 1/2 cup chopped fresh basil
» 1/2 cup chopped marjoram or oregano
» 28 ounces diced canned tomatoes, or 12 fresh plum tomatoes, chopped
» 1/4 teaspoon fine sea salt
» Freshly ground pepper

1. In a 4-quart saucepan, add olive oil and heat to medium.

2. Add garlic and cook until fragrant. When garlic becomes fragrant, add basil, oregano, and tomatoes. Simmer 20 minutes. (See Cook's Tip: If meatballs are to be added, you can add them at this point.)

3. Add sea salt and pepper. Add more basil if desired. Simmer 10 minutes more or longer, if time permits.

COOK'S TIP:
This sauce is suitable for pizza and pasta sauces, and it's great with meatballs. You can also drizzle this over a meatloaf 15 minutes before the meatloaf is finished baking.

Exchanges/Choices		
2 Vegetable	Calories 105	Potassium 440 mg
1 1/2 Fat	Calories from Fat 65	Total Carbohydrate 10 g
	Total Fat 7.0 g	Dietary Fiber 3 g
	Saturated Fat 1.0 g	Sugars 5 g
	Trans Fat 0.0 g	Protein 2 g
	Cholesterol 0 mg	Phosphorus 50 mg
	Sodium 430 mg	

Orecchiette with Pancetta and Zucchini

SERVES: 4 / SERVING SIZE: 1/4 RECIPE

This dish is reminiscent of one that I enjoyed in Soave, Italy. Naturally, you will want to pair it with an Italian Soave. Pancetta is an Italian "bacon" that is not smoked. It's readily available in the grocery store.

» 1/2 pound orecchiette pasta
» 1 tablespoon extra virgin olive oil
» 4 ounces pancetta, finely diced
» 2 cloves garlic, peeled and minced
» 2 cups zucchini, halved and sliced thinly
» 1/2 cup low-sodium chicken stock
» 1/2 teaspoon fine sea salt
» 1/8 teaspoon freshly cracked black pepper

1. Cook pasta to al dente stage in a large pot of boiling water. Drain and set aside.

2. Place olive oil and pancetta in large sauté pan. Cook until pancetta begins to brown. Add garlic and zucchini. Cook just until zucchini begins to become tender, about 2 minutes.

3. Add chicken stock, salt, and pepper. Cook until chicken stock is heated. Add pasta and mix well. (A little more olive oil or chicken stock can be added if you like your pasta dishes a little saucier.)

Exchanges/Choices		
3 Starch	Calories 305	Potassium 375 mg
1 1/2 Fat	Calories from Fat 80	Total Carbohydrate 45 g
	Total Fat 9.0 g	Dietary Fiber 2 g
	Saturated Fat 2.2 g	Sugars 3 g
	Trans Fat 0.0 g	Protein 11 g
	Cholesterol 10 mg	Phosphorus 205 mg
	Sodium 430 mg	

Pasta with Lemon, Pepper, and Fresh Herbs

SERVES: 8 / SERVING SIZE: 1/8 RECIPE

This dish is great for buffets and picnics as it can be served at room temperature and nothing will spoil. It is also very refreshing for warmer weather.

» 1 pound linguine, cooked al dente
» 2 cloves garlic, sliced thin
» 1/3 cup extra virgin olive oil
» Sea salt
» Freshly ground black pepper
» 2–3 lemons, juiced
» 1/2 cup roughly chopped fresh herbs
   (Italian parsley, basil, or chives)

1. Cook pasta according to package directions.

2. Slice garlic and place in sauté pan. Add oil and heat until fragrant and garlic is light to golden brown. Transfer to a heatproof bowl or 4 cup Pyrex measuring cup. Add 2 pinches sea salt and a few grindings of fresh pepper. Add juice of 1 1/2–2 lemons. Whisk together until creamy.

3. Pour mixture over cooked pasta and toss well. Add fresh herbs and additional lemon slices, if desired. Serve hot or at room temperature.

Exchanges/Choices		
3 Starch	Calories 305	Potassium 85 mg
1 1/2 Fat	Calories from Fat 90	Total Carbohydrate 44 g
	Total Fat 10.0 g	Dietary Fiber 3 g
	Saturated Fat 1.5 g	Sugars 1 g
	Trans Fat 0.0 g	Protein 8 g
	Cholesterol 0 mg	Phosphorus 85 mg
	Sodium 45 mg	

Porcini Mushroom Sauce for Pasta

SERVES: 6 / SERVING SIZE: 1/6 RECIPE

Porcini and portobello mushrooms give your dishes a very "meaty," flavor so this is a great way to enjoy an occasional meatless meal.

» 1 ounce dried porcini or portobello mushrooms, roughly chopped
» 1 tablespoon extra virgin olive oil
» 1 medium onion, chopped
» 2 cloves garlic, minced
» 2 portobello mushroom caps
» 1/2 cup dry red wine
» 28 ounces crushed tomatoes
» 1/2 cup fresh basil leaves
» 1 tablespoon fresh oregano leaves

{ COOK'S TIP:
You can also use a slow-cooker to make this recipe. Just cook on low for 8 hours, or on high for 4 hours. }

1. Bring a small pan of water to a boil and add dried mushrooms. Steep for 5 minutes. Drain and save liquid.

2. Place olive oil in 6-quart saucepan. Add onion and garlic. Cook until onion is translucent and garlic is fragrant, about 2–3 minutes. Do not brown the garlic. Add mushrooms and continue cooking.

3. Add wine. Deglaze pan. Add mushroom steeping liquid and tomatoes.

4. Simmer for 30 minutes or longer. Garnish with basil leaves and oregano before serving.

Exchanges/Choices	Calories 100	Potassium 615 mg
3 Vegetable	Calories from Fat 25	Total Carbohydrate 17 g
1/2 Fat	Total Fat 3.0 g	Dietary Fiber 4 g
	Saturated Fat 0.4 g	Sugars 7 g
	Trans Fat 0.0 g	Protein 4 g
	Cholesterol 0 mg	Phosphorus 90 mg
	Sodium 180 mg	

Buffalo Mushroom Sauce for Pasta

SERVES: 6 / SERVING SIZE: 1/6 RECIPE

Buffalo has little to no saturated fat, which makes it heart healthy. The addition of the mushrooms adds to the richness of the flavor of the buffalo.

» 1 ounce dried porcini, roughly chopped
» 1 tablespoon extra virgin olive oil
» 1 medium onion, chopped
» 2 cloves garlic, minced
» 1 pound ground buffalo, or lean ground beef
» 1/2 cup dry red wine
» 28 ounces crushed tomatoes
» 1/2 cup fresh basil leaves
» 1 tablespoon fresh oregano leaves

1. Bring a small pan of water to a boil and add dried mushrooms. Steep for 5 minutes. Drain and save liquid.

2. Place extra virgin olive oil in 6-quart saucepan. Add onion and garlic. Cook until onion is translucent and garlic is fragrant. Do not brown the garlic. Add meat and cook until nicely browned.

3. Add wine. Deglaze pan. Add mushroom steeping liquid, tomatoes, basil, and oregano.

4. Simmer for 60 minutes or longer. Garnish with basil and oregano before serving.

{ COOK'S TIP: }
You can use a slow-cooker to make this recipe. Just cook on low for 8 hours, or on high for 4 hours.

Exchanges/Choices		
3 Vegetable	Calories 200	Potassium 775 mg
2 Lean Meat	Calories from Fat 35	Total Carbohydrate 17 g
1/2 Fat	Total Fat 4.0 g	Dietary Fiber 4 g
	Saturated Fat 0.9 g	Sugars 8 g
	Trans Fat 0.0 g	Protein 20 g
	Cholesterol 50 mg	Phosphorus 195 mg
	Sodium 210 mg	

Penne with Artichokes, Asparagus & Tomato

SERVES: 8 / SERVING SIZE: 1/8 RECIPE

I developed this recipe for a class I was teaching called "Meatless Italian." The cheeses will provide some protein.

» 1 pound whole-grain penne pasta

» 2 tablespoons extra virgin olive oil

» 3 large garlic cloves, minced

» 28 ounces San Marzano tomatoes

» 1/4 cup fresh basil leaves

» 2 tablespoons chopped fresh Italian parsley

» 1/2 teaspoon fine sea salt

» 1/2 teaspoon freshly ground black pepper

» 2 10-ounce boxes frozen artichoke hearts, or 1 recipe braised artichokes (page 101)

» 1 pound asparagus spears, lightly steamed until fork tender, cut into 1-inch pieces

» 1 1/2 cups fresh ricotta cheese

» 1 ounce piece of Parmigiano-Reggiano cheese, grated (for garnish)

1. Cook pasta, according to package directions, in large pot of boiling water. Cook until al dente. Drain and set aside.

2. Place olive oil in large saucepan. Add garlic and heat until garlic is light golden brown. Add tomatoes, basil, parsley, salt, and pepper. Bring to a boil and stir to mix well. Add artichokes and asparagus and simmer.

3. Place 3 tablespoon of fresh ricotta in each pasta bowl. Pour pasta over the ricotta and garnish with Parmigiano-Reggiano. Serve immediately.

Exchanges/Choices	Calories 370	Potassium 555 mg
3 Starch	Calories from Fat 90	Total Carbohydrate 58 g
2 Vegetable	Total Fat 10.0 g	Dietary Fiber 11 g
1 Med-Fat Meat	Saturated Fat 3.6 g	Sugars 6 g
1/2 Fat	Trans Fat 0.0 g	Protein 17 g
	Cholesterol 15 mg	Phosphorus 290 mg
	Sodium 420 mg	

Lentils with Italian Turkey Sausage

SERVES: 6 / SERVING SIZE: 1/6 RECIPE

The first time I prepared this on the set of "Stress Free Cooking," the crew loved it and requested it every season.

» 1 pound good quality Italian turkey sausage (either hot or sweet)
» 1 tablespoon olive oil
» 1 medium onion, chopped (about 1 cup)
» 2 cloves garlic, peeled and minced
» 1/4 teaspoon dried oregano
» 1 medium carrot, quartered and sliced thin (about 1/2 cup)
» 1 stalk celery, sliced thin (about 1/2 cup)
» 1 cup dried Italian lentils
» 4–5 cups chicken or vegetable stock
» Fresh chopped herbs such as basil or Italian parsley
» Grana Padano cheese, grated (or any cheese you like)

1. Remove casing from sausage and break into small pieces with your fingers. Set aside.

2. Thinly film a sauté pan with extra virgin olive oil. Add onion and garlic and cook 2–3 minutes, until onion begins to soften. Clear a small space in the pan and add the oregano.

3. Add sausage and cook until sausage is browned. Add carrots, celery, and lentils and toss well with sausage mixture. Add 2 cups stock and cook until most of the stock is evaporated. Add more stock, 1 cup at a time until lentils are tender, approximately 30 minutes.

4. Garnish with chopped herbs and a sprinkling of grated cheese.

{ COOK'S TIP:
This can easily become a vegetarian dish by leaving out the sausage and using vegtable stock. }

Exchanges/Choices		
1 Starch	Calories 260	Potassium 690 mg
1 Vegetable	Calories from Fat 90	Total Carbohydrate 22 g
2 Med-Fat Meat	Total Fat 10.0 g	Dietary Fiber 8 g
	Saturated Fat 2.3 g	Sugars 4 g
	Trans Fat 0.2 g	Protein 22 g
	Cholesterol 45 mg	Phosphorus 280 mg
	Sodium 550 mg	

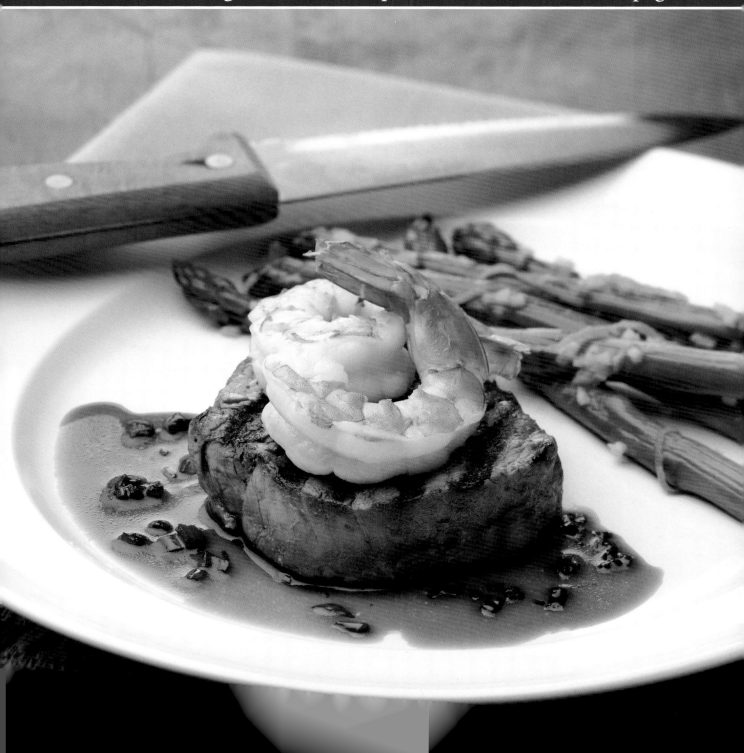

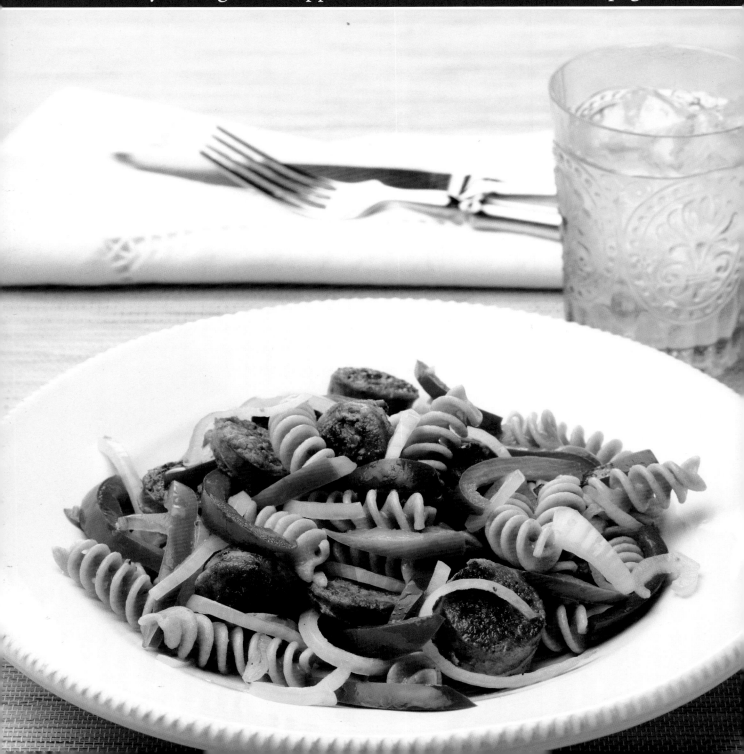

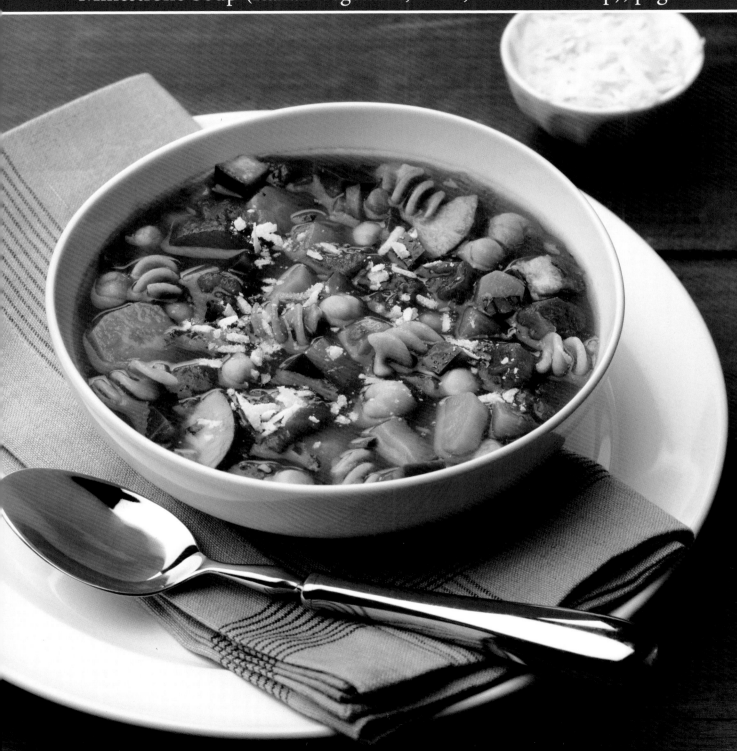

Minestrone Soup (Italian Vegetable, Bean, and Pasta Soup), page 68

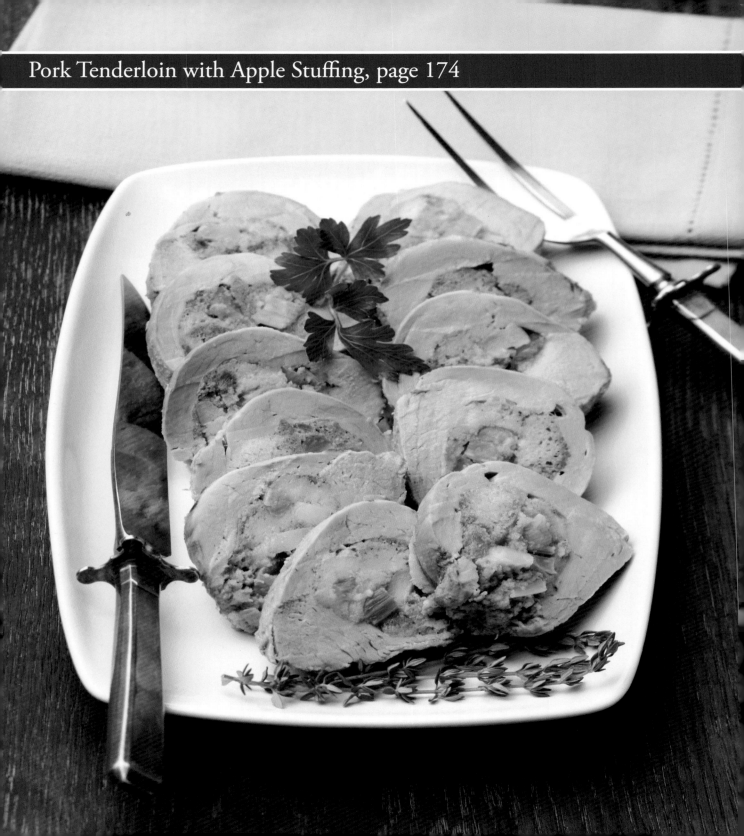

Pork Tenderloin with Apple Stuffing, page 174

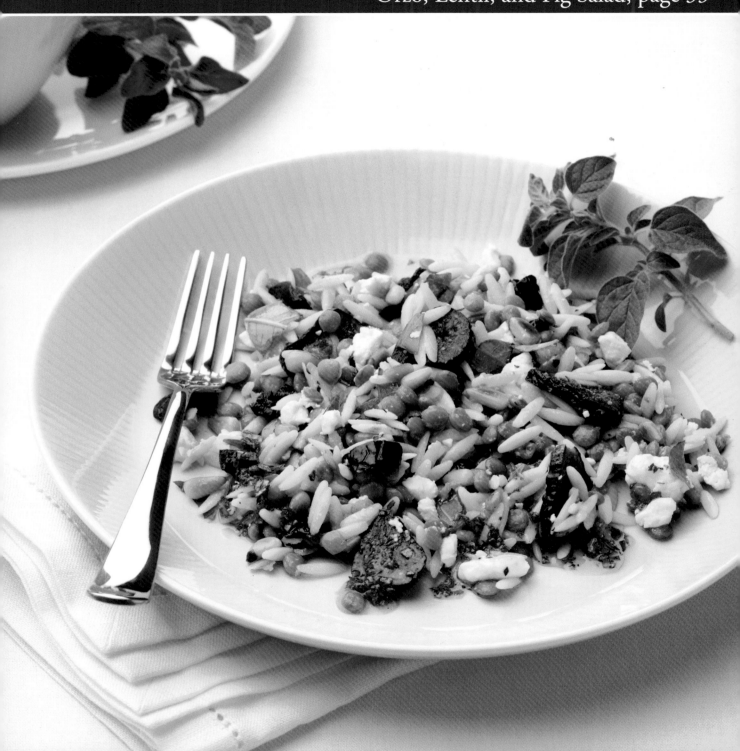

Orzo, Lentil, and Fig Salad, page 33

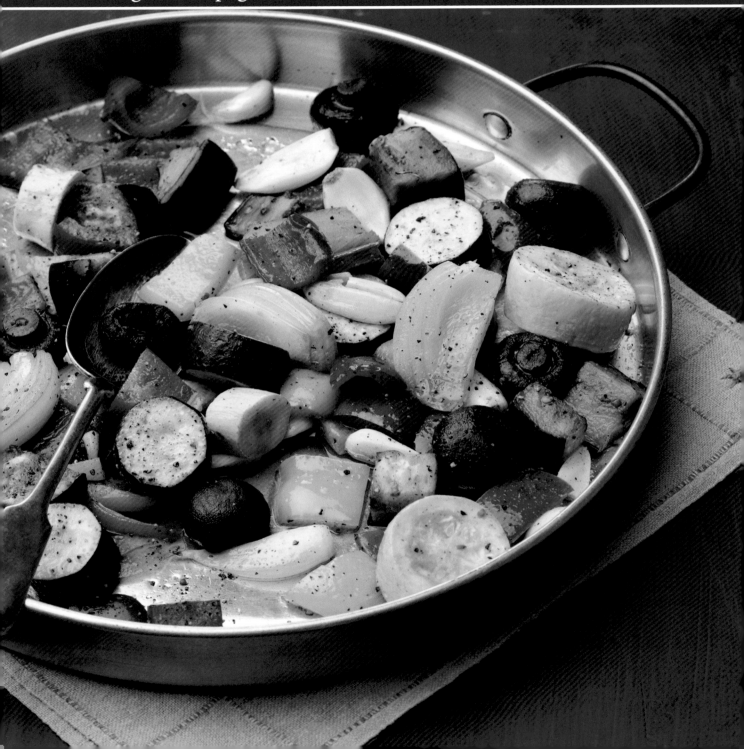
Roasted Vegetables, page 104

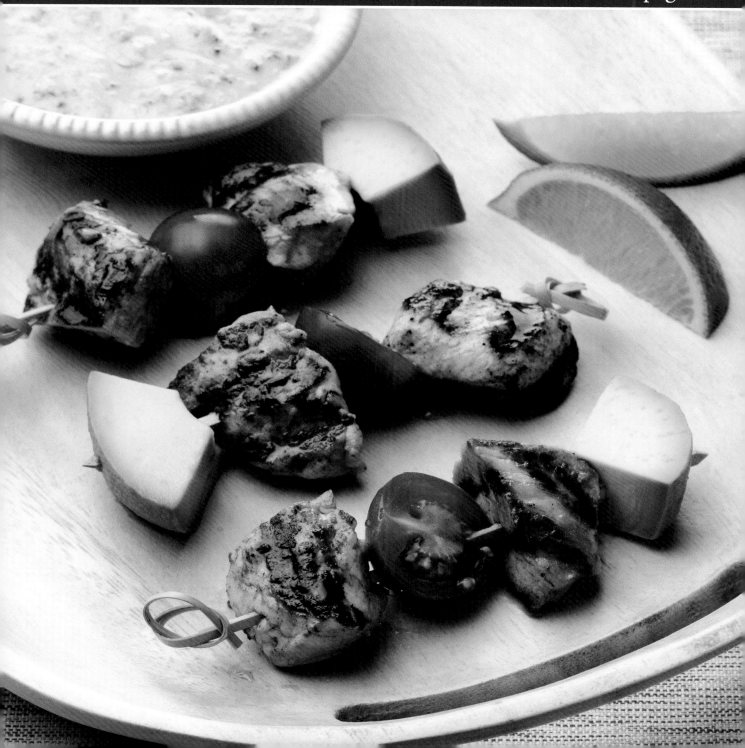

Turkey Kebabs with Avocado & Tomato, page 28

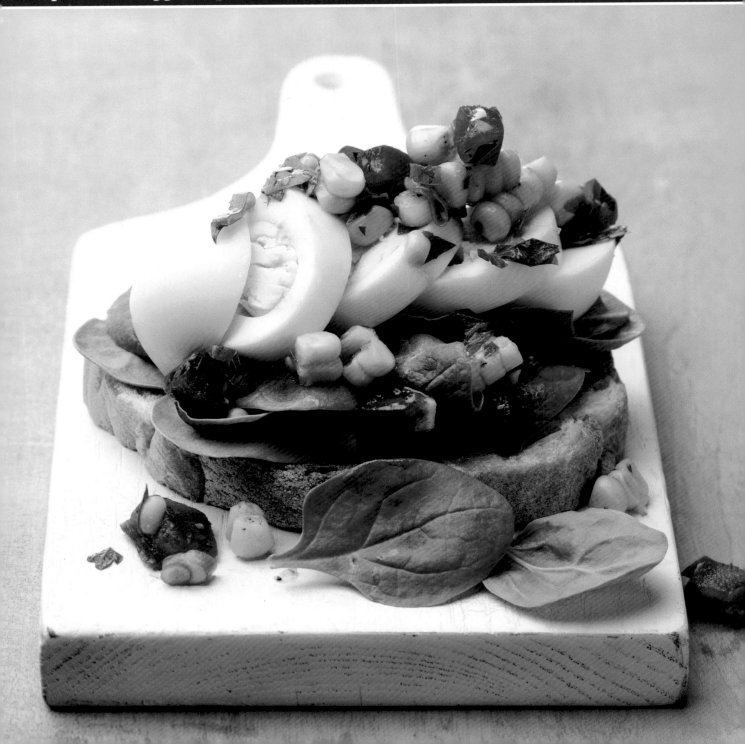

Risotto Style Fregula (Sardinian Toasted Pasta)

SERVES: 4 / SERVING SIZE: 1/4 RECIPE

Fregula is ancient Sardinian pasta that is very flavorful and cooks quickly. I love the toasty, nutty flavor and variety that it adds to my dishes.

» 4–6 cups low-sodium chicken or vegetable stock
» 1 cup dry white wine
» 1 tablespoon extra virgin olive oil
» 2 shallots, minced
» 1 clove garlic, minced
» 1 cup uncooked fregula pasta
» 1/4 cup finely minced Italian parsley
» 3 Tablespoons finely grated Parmigiano-Reggiano cheese, or mixed Italian cheeses
» Fine sea salt
» Freshly ground black pepper

1. Place stock and wine in small saucepan and heat to simmering.

2. Place olive oil in 4-quart pan. Warm the oil and add the shallots and garlic. Cook until fragrant and shallots are translucent. Add pasta. Add stock one cup at a time, adding when each cup has been absorbed by the pasta.

3. Cook until fregula is tender. (You can add additional stock if you like your risotto-style fregula with more liquid.)

4. Stir in parsley and cheese. Season with salt and pepper to taste. Serve.

Exchanges/Choices	Calories 235	Potassium 345 mg
2 1/2 Starch	Calories from Fat 45	Total Carbohydrate 36 g
1 Fat	Total Fat 5.0 g	Dietary Fiber 2 g
	Saturated Fat 1.4 g	Sugars 3 g
	Trans Fat 0.0 g	Protein 9 g
	Cholesterol 5 mg	Phosphorus 140 mg
	Sodium 115 mg	

Roasted Vegetable Quinoa Strudel with Warm Shallot Vinaigrette

SERVES: 6 / SERVING SIZE: 1/6 RECIPE

Quinoa (keen-wah) is a high protein grain and an ancient cousin to Amaranth. It is very tiny and has a nutty flavor.

Strudel

» 2 cloves garlic, peeled and thinly sliced
» 3 cups chopped fresh vegetables, such as zucchini, mushrooms, red bell pepper, and onion
» 1 1/2 tablespoons olive oil
» 2 cups cooked quinoa, cooked according to package
» 1/2 cup chopped basil
» 1/4 cup freshly grated Parmigiano-Reggiano cheese
» 6 sheets (14 × 18-inch piece) frozen or fresh phyllo pastry (see Cook's Tip)
» Nonstick cooking spray

Warm Shallot Vinaigrette

» 3 tablespoons olive oil
» 2 tablespoons white wine vinegar
» 2 teaspoons honey
» 1 chopped shallot

1. Preheat oven to 425°F.

2. Place garlic and vegetables on sheet pan lined with parchment paper and toss with small amount of olive oil. Bake for 30 minutes. Cool. Mix vegetables with quinoa. Add basil and Parmigiano-Reggiano.

3. Lay phyllo out near your work surface and cover with a damp towel. Take one sheet of phyllo and lay it on top of a baking sheet. Spray with cooking spray. Repeat this process with the rest of the phyllo sheets.

4. Spread vegetable mixture over dough leaving a 2-inch edge all around. Fold in short sides and begin rolling like a jellyroll. Place seam side down on baking sheet. Spray again with cooking spray. Wipe excess from baking sheet.

(Continued on next page)

Exchanges/Choices		
2 Starch	Calories 260	Potassium 305 mg
1 Vegetable	Calories from Fat 100	Total Carbohydrate 35 g
2 Fat	Total Fat 11.0 g	Dietary Fiber 3 g
	Saturated Fat 2.0 g	Sugars 6 g
	Trans Fat 0.0 g	Protein 6 g
	Cholesterol 5 mg	Phosphorus 160 mg
	Sodium 120 mg	

(Roasted Vegetable Quinoa Strudel with Warm Shallot Vinaigrette Continued)

5. Turn oven down to 400°F and bake for 30 minutes or until golden brown and beautiful.

6. In the meantime, Heat olive oil in a small sauté pan. Add white wine vinegar, honey, and shallot. Mix well and keep warm. Drizzle over Strudel.

{ COOK'S TIP:
Defrost frozen phyllo in the
refrigerator for at least 3 hours or
overnight. }

Risotto with Porcini Mushrooms

SERVES: 6 / SERVING SIZE: 1/6 RECIPE

The key to good risotto is the slow absorption of the hot liquid, which can take 20–40 minutes. Try not to rush this dish.

» 1 1/2 cups dry white wine
» 4 cups low-sodium chicken or mushroom stock
» 1 cup dried porcini, rehydrated
» 1 teaspoon extra virgin olive oil
» 1 cup onion, chopped
» 2 cups carnaroli or arborio rice, checked over for imperfect grains
» 1/2 teaspoon fine sea salt
» 1/2 teaspoon freshly ground pepper
» 1/2 cup freshly grated Parmigiano-Reggiano cheese
» 2 tablespoons finely minced Italian parsley

{ **VARIATION:**
Add sautéed chicken, cut into bite-size pieces, along with the porcini. }

1. In a 4-quart saucepan, bring wine and stock to a boil and keep simmering on stove. Add porcini and simmer 5 minutes. Drain this mixture through a coffee filter. Reserve porcini and chop into bite-size pieces. Place stock and wine back in pan and simmer.

2. Using a heavy, 5-quart saucepan or chef's pan, thinly film the pan with olive oil and add onion. Sauté until onion starts to soften. Add rice, salt, and pepper and coat rice grains with olive oil mixture. Add stock mixture 1 cup at a time and stir until each addition of liquid is absorbed.

3. After last addition of stock is absorbed, add Parmigiano-Reggiano cheese. When all of the stock is absorbed—which can take anywhere from 20–40 minutes—and rice grains are creamy, you can add the parsley and porcini. Serve immediately!

Exchanges/Choices		
3 Starch	Calories 280	Potassium 310 mg
1 Vegetable	Calories from Fat 25	Total Carbohydrate 52 g
1/2 Fat	Total Fat 3.0 g	Dietary Fiber 3 g
	Saturated Fat 1.5 g	Sugars 2 g
	Trans Fat 0.0 g	Protein 8 g
	Cholesterol 10 mg	Phosphorus 145 mg
	Sodium 295 mg	

Macaroni and Cheese

SERVES: 8 / SERVING SIZE: 1/8 RECIPE

Everyone loves Macaroni and Cheese. It's simple to make and freezes well. Using low-fat diary products helps lighten this dish. My kids always loved their Grandma's mac & cheese so I created this lighter version for them.

» 1/2 pound whole-wheat pasta (shape of your choice)
» 1 1/3 tablespoons unsalted butter
» 1/4 cup flour
» 2 1/2 cups skim milk
» 6 ounces shredded Cabot 75% reduced-fat cheddar cheese, reserving 1/4 cup for topping
» 1/2 teaspoon fine sea salt
» 1/4 teaspoon freshly ground white or black pepper

{ COOK'S TIP:
Mix chopped, fresh herbs into the cheese sauce. Add 1/4 cup bread crumbs and diced prosciutto to the cheese before sprinkling on top. }

1. Cook pasta, according to directions, to al dente stage. Drain and set aside. (Remember to cook pasta in at least 4–6 quarts water. Cooking it in too little water will result in sticky, gummy pasta.)

2. Preheat oven to 375°F. In a 4-quart saucepan, melt butter and whisk in flour. (The mixture will be dry.) Cook over medium heat for 2 minutes and add half the milk. Whisk until smooth. Add remaining milk and whisk again until smooth. Cook until thickened, approximately 3–5 minutes.

3. Remove pan from heat. Gradually add cheese 1/4 cup at a time, whisking until smooth. Season with salt and pepper.

4. Mix cheese sauce with pasta and place in 9-inch square casserole dish. Top with additional grated cheese. Bake until casserole bubbles and cheese topping is melted, about 25–30 minutes.

Exchanges/Choices		
1 1/2 Starch	Calories 200	Potassium 185 mg
1/2 Fat-Free Milk	Calories from Fat 40	Total Carbohydrate 28 g
1 Lean Meat	Total Fat 4.5 g	Dietary Fiber 2 g
	Saturated Fat 2.5 g	Sugars 5 g
	Trans Fat 0.0 g	Protein 14 g
	Cholesterol 15 mg	Phosphorus 255 mg
	Sodium 330 mg	

Whole-Wheat Pizza or Bread Dough

SERVES: 12 OR 16 / SERVING SIZE: 1 SLICE OR 1 ROLL

This recipe will yield one large pizza that will serve 12 or 16 dinner rolls.

» 1 1/2 cups all-purpose flour
» 1 1/2 cups white-wheat flour
» 1 tablespoon active yeast
» 1 teaspoon fine sea salt
» 1–1 1/2 cups tepid water (water between 110–120°F)
» 1 teaspoon extra virgin olive oil

1. Place all dry ingredients in the bowl of your food processor. Pulse a few times to blend well.

2. With the machine running, add 1 cup of water in a slow and steady stream. The dough should form a ball. If it seems too dry, add more water, 1 tablespoon at a time. (The dough is perfect when it is no longer sticky and feels smooth. If it is too sticky or wet, you can more flour 1 tablespoon at a time.)

3. Place dough in a large bowl with olive oil. Cover dough completely with oil and then cover tightly with plastic wrap and a cloth towel.

4. Let rise in a warm place for at least 1 hour. (I usually place it in the oven with the oven off and the oven light on.)

(Continued on next page)

(Whole-Wheat Pizza or Bread Dough Continued)

5. After the dough doubles in size, punch it down and let it rise again for as long as possible, at least 1 hour.

(Analysis for pizza)
Exchanges/Choices
1 1/2 Starch

Calories 125
   Calories from Fat 10
Total Fat 1.0 g
   Saturated Fat 0.1 g
   Trans Fat 0.0 g
Cholesterol 0 mg
Sodium 200 mg

Potassium 100 mg
Total Carbohydrate 24 g
   Dietary Fiber 3 g
   Sugars 0 g
Protein 4 g
Phosphorus 80 mg

(Analysis for rolls)
Exchanges/Choices
1 Starch

Calories 95
   Calories from Fat 5
Total Fat 0.5 g
   Saturated Fat 0.1 g
   Trans Fat 0.0 g
Cholesterol 0 mg
Sodium 150 mg

Potassium 75 mg
Total Carbohydrate 18 g
   Dietary Fiber 2 g
   Sugars 0 g
Protein 3 g
Phosphorus 60 mg

CHAPTER 8:
Poultry

The Stress Free Diabetes Kitchen

Poultry

Cornish Hens Stuffed with Potatoes, Capers, and Garlic

SERVES: 4 / SERVING SIZE: 1/2 HEN

I love Cornish Hens for entertaining—they are easy, impressive, and delicious!

» 2 pounds baby Yukon Gold potatoes, baked or microwaved until fork tender, cut into 1-inch pieces
» 2 tablespoons capers
» 2 tablespoons chopped flat leaf parsley
» 2 cloves garlic, minced
» 1 tablespoon extra virgin olive oil
» 1/2 teaspoon fine sea salt
» 1/2 teaspoon coarsely ground black pepper
» 2 Cornish hens (3 1/2–4 pounds total)

1. Preheat oven to 400°F.

2. In a large bowl, mix together the potatoes, capers, parsley, garlic, olive oil, salt, and pepper.

3. Wash and dry the hens. Stuff hens with potato mixture. Sprinkle outside of hens with salt and pepper.

4. Place on roasting rack or parchment-lined baking sheet. Roast for approximately 1 hour. Remove skin before serving.

Exchanges/Choices	Calories 470	Potassium 1270 mg
3 Starch	Calories from Fat 100	Total Carbohydrate 44 g
5 Lean Meat	Total Fat 11.0 g	Dietary Fiber 4 g
	Saturated Fat 2.4 g	Sugars 2 g
	Trans Fat 0.0 g	Protein 48 g
	Cholesterol 200 mg	Phosphorus 465 mg
	Sodium 555 mg	

Turkey Breast Stuffed with Fresh Herbs & Garlic

SERVES: 12 / SERVING SIZE: 1/12 RECIPE

This turkey breast is wonderful, and the leftovers can be used in so many other dishes. You can ask your butcher to de-bone the turkey breast for you.

» 1 turkey breast (about 7 pounds, before boning), boned with skin on
» 1 1/2 cups of your favorite herbs (basil, parsley, rosemary, and thyme), roughly chopped
» 4 cloves garlic, minced
» 1/2 teaspoon fine sea salt
» 1/2 teaspoon freshly ground black pepper
» 1 teaspoon extra virgin olive oil
» Additional salt and pepper (optional)

1. Preheat oven to 375°F.

2. Lay turkey breast skin side down on a cutting board. Pound or cut into the flesh to make it as even a thickness as possible. It won't be perfectly flat.

3. Sprinkle with herbs, garlic, salt, and pepper. Roll turkey breast and tie with twine. Rub the outside with extra virgin olive oil and sprinkle again with salt and pepper, if desired.

4. Place turkey breast on a parchment-lined baking sheet and roast for 50–60 minutes, or until a meat thermometer registers 155–160°F. Remove from oven and let rest for 10–15 minutes. (Letting it rest makes slicing easier.) Remove skin before eating.

Exchanges/Choices
6 Lean Meat

Calories 235
  Calories from Fat 15
Total Fat 1.5 g
  Saturated Fat 0.5 g
  Trans Fat 0.0 g
Cholesterol 140 mg
Sodium 185 mg

Potassium 515 mg
Total Carbohydrate 1 g
  Dietary Fiber 0 g
  Sugars 0 g
Protein 50 g
Phosphorus 380 mg

Bloody Mary Cornish Hens

SERVES: 4 / SERVING SIZE: 1/4 RECIPE

This is a "fun" recipe that can be cooked on the grill or in your oven. I was inspired to create this recipe when there was Bloody Mary mix leftover after a party. This dish is great served with couscous cooked in chicken stock.

» 2 Cornish hens (about 3–3 1/2 pounds)
» 2 cups tomato juice
» 1/2 cup roughly chopped Italian parsley
» 6 garlic cloves, sliced into rounds
» 1 teaspoon celery salt
» 1 tablespoon Worcestershire sauce
» 1/4 cup vodka
» Juice of 1 lemon
» 1 tablespoon horseradish
» 1/2 teaspoon freshly ground peppercorns
» 1 tablespoon extra virgin olive oil

1. Wash hens and remove any visible fat. Cut hens into two halves.

2. Mix together tomato juice, parsley, garlic, celery salt, Worcestershire sauce, vodka, lemon juice, horseradish, pepper, and olive oil. Marinate hens for 30 minutes or overnight.

3. Preheat grill. Brush grill to ensure clean surface. Place hens skin side up on grill and grill on medium with lid closed, about 30–40 minutes or until it reaches an internal temperature of 165°F. Remove skin before eating.

COOK'S TIP:

If you don't have a grill, place hens on parchment-lined baking sheet and bake at 400°F for 45 minutes to 1 hour. If using convection oven, bake at 375°F for 45 minutes.

Exchanges/Choices	Calories 250	Potassium 585 mg
1/2 Carbohydrate	Calories from Fat 70	Total Carbohydrate 5 g
5 Lean Meat	Total Fat 8.0 g	Dietary Fiber 1 g
	Saturated Fat 1.8 g	Sugars 3 g
	Trans Fat 0.0 g	Protein 37 g
	Cholesterol 165 mg	Phosphorus 250 mg
	Sodium 370 mg	

Chicken Parmigiano

SERVES: 10 / SERVING SIZE: 1/10 RECIPE

Quick Marinara Sauce
- » 1 teaspoon extra virgin olive oil
- » 2 cloves garlic, chopped
- » 2 cans (28 ounces each) tomato purée or crushed tomatoes
- » 1 cup fresh basil leaves

Chicken
- » 4 boneless, skinless chicken breasts (about 1 1/2 pounds)
- » 3 large eggs
- » 1 cup Italian-Style bread crumbs
- » 1/4 cup grated Parmigiano-Reggiano cheese
- » 1 teaspoon salt
- » 1/2 teaspoon black pepper
- » 1 tablespoon extra virgin olive oil
- » 1 pound spaghetti or pasta of your choice
- » 10 teaspoons part-skim mozzarella cheese

1. Preheat oven to 375°F. Place a little olive oil in the bottom of a large saucepan (just enough to cover the bottom). Add garlic and cook until fragrant but not dark brown. Add tomatoes and basil. Bring to a low boil and then turn down to simmer while you prepare the chicken.

2. Pound chicken breast to even thickness of about 1/2 inch.

3. In a large dish or pie plate, scramble eggs. In a separate dish or pie plate, combine bread crumbs, parmesan cheese, salt, and pepper and mix well.

4. Dip chicken in egg, and then dip in bread crumb mixture. Place on parchment paper or aluminum foil until ready to cook.

(Continued on next page)

Exchanges/Choices
3 starch
2 Vegetable
2 Lean Meat
1/2 Fat

Calories 400
   Calories from Fat 65
Total Fat 7.0 g
   Saturated Fat 2.1 g
   Trans Fat 0.0 g
Cholesterol 100 mg
Sodium 535 mg

Potassium 940 mg
Total Carbohydrate 57 g
   Dietary Fiber 5 g
   Sugars 9 g
Protein 27 g
Phosphorus 305 mg

(Chicken Parmigiano Continued)

5. Place some marinara in the bottom of the baking dish. Set aside while cooking the chicken.

6. Place enough olive oil in the sauté or frying pan to lightly cover the bottom. Turn pan to medium-high and let it heat up. Add chicken breast and cook until golden on each side, about 3 minutes per side.

7. Place chicken in baking dish. When all the chicken is cooked, cover with more marinara and top each piece of chicken with 1 teaspoon shredded mozzarella cheese. Bake 25–30 minutes until sauce is bubbly and cheese is melted.

8. Serve with pasta and remaining marinara sauce. Sprinkle each serving with 1 teaspoon mozzarella.

Chicken or Turkey Pot Pie

SERVES: 6 / SERVING SIZE: 1/6 RECIPE

Comfort food can be enjoyed even if you want to cook healthier. Phyllo dough makes a fabulously crispy top crust without the fat. Garlic mashed potatoes (page 123) make a great alternative top "crust."

» 2 tablespoons extra virgin olive oil, divided use
» 1/2 cup chopped onion
» 1 clove garlic, minced
» 1 cup sliced celery
» 1 cup carrot, sliced 1/4-inch thick
» 1 tablespoon unsalted butter
» 1/4 cup all-purpose flour
» 2 cups low-sodium chicken stock, plus additional, if desired
» 3 cups poached chicken or turkey, or leftover chicken or turkey
» 1 cup frozen baby peas
» 2 tablespoons chopped Italian parsley
» 1/2 teaspoon fine sea salt
» 1/2 teaspoon freshly ground pepper
» 5–6 sheets (14 × 18-inch) thawed phyllo dough
» olive oil mister

1. Preheat oven to 375°F.

2. Place 1 tablespoon olive oil in saucepan. Add onion and garlic and cook 2–3 minutes until it begins to soften. Add celery and carrot and cook 5 minutes to soften. Set aside.

3. Place 1 tablespoon of olive oil and butter in 4-quart saucepan. Melt butter. Whisk in flour and mix well. (Mixture will be dry.) Gradually add 1 cup stock to saucepan. Cook 2–3 minutes until mixture begins to thicken and takes on a golden color.

(Continued on next page)

Exchanges/Choices		
1 starch	Calories 280	Potassium 380 mg
1 Vegetable	Calories from Fat 90	Total Carbohydrate 23 g
3 Lean Meat	Total Fat 10.0 g	Dietary Fiber 3 g
1 Fat	Saturated Fat 2.6 g	Sugars 3 g
	Trans Fat 0.0 g	Protein 25 g
	Cholesterol 60 mg	Phosphorus 180 mg
	Sodium 390 mg	

(Chicken Parmigiano Contined)

4. Add chicken, peas, parsley, and additional stock to achieve desired consistency (some like it soupy, some like it thick). Season with salt and pepper to taste. Place mixture in baking dish.

5. Spray each sheet of phyllo with olive oil mister and place on top of baking dish. Trim edges.

6. Bake for approximately 25 minutes or until crust is golden and pie is bubbly.

{
COOK'S TIP:
» Flour mixture must be cooked at least 2–3 minutes to lose the uncooked flour taste.
» Pie plate can be sprayed with nonstick cooking spray or lightly buttered.
}

Chicken with Portobello Mushroom Sauce

SERVES: 8 / SERVING SIZE: 1/8 RECIPE

A great dish that is both easy and elegant.

» 4 boneless, skinless, chicken breasts (about 1 1/2 pounds)
» 4 egg whites
» Fine sea salt
» Freshly ground pepper
» 2 cups dry bread crumbs, unseasoned
» 1/2 cup Parmigiano-Reggiano cheese, finely grated
» 1 tablespoon extra virgin olive oil
» 2–3 large portobello mushrooms (about 2 cups sliced)
» 1 cup dry white wine (such as Orvieto or Pinot Grigio)
» 1 cup low-sodium chicken stock

1. Pound chicken breasts to 1/2-inch even thickness.

2. In a small bowl, scramble eggs whites with a pinch of salt and a few grindings of pepper.

3. Mix bread crumbs with cheese and place on foil or parchment.

4. Dip chicken in egg mixture and then in bread crumbs. You can press the mixture onto the chicken with your hands to ensure even coating. Set aside.

5. Heat sauté pan and thinly film with olive oil. When oil is hot, add chicken and brown until golden on each side. Add sliced mushrooms to pan surface and cook 5 minutes. Add wine and stock and simmer 5 minutes more.

Exchanges/Choices
1 Starch
5 Lean Meat

Calories 315
  Calories from Fat 55
Total Fat 6.0 g
  Saturated Fat 1.8 g
  Trans Fat 0.0 g
Cholesterol 55 mg
Sodium 540 mg

Potassium 595 mg
Total Carbohydrate 17 g
  Dietary Fiber 1 g
  Sugars 3 g
Protein 42 g
Phosphorus 245 mg

Italian Turkey Sausage and Peppers over Whole-Wheat Pasta

SERVES: 8 / SERVING SIZE: 1/8 RECIPE

» 1 pound whole-wheat pasta (any shape you like)
» 1 teaspoon salt
» 1 pound hot Italian turkey sausage (sweet will also work), sliced into 1/2-inch thick discs
» 1 clove garlic, minced
» 2 medium bell peppers, thinly sliced
» 1 large onion, thinly sliced
» 1/4 teaspoon fine sea salt
» 1/4 teaspoon freshly ground pepper

1. Cook pasta according to package instructions. Add salt to pasta water before cooking.

2. Heat sauté pan and add sausage, garlic, peppers, and onions. Cook until sausage is no longer pink and peppers and onions are tender.

3. Toss pasta with sausage mixture. Season with salt and pepper and serve.

Exchanges/Choices
3 Starch
1 Vegetable
1 Med-Fat Meat

Calories 330
  Calories from Fat 65
Total Fat 7.0 g
  Saturated Fat 1.7 g
  Trans Fat 0.0 g
Cholesterol 35 mg
Sodium 535 mg

Potassium 315 mg
Total Carbohydrate 50 g
  Dietary Fiber 7 g
  Sugars 4 g
Protein 17 g
Phosphorus 220 mg

Lemon Chicken with Capers

SERVES: 4 / SERVING SIZE: 1/4 RECIPE

If you love lemons and capers you must make this dish.

» 1/2 cup Wondra flour
» Pinch fine sea salt
» Freshly ground pepper
» 1 tablespoon extra virgin olive oil
» 4 boneless, skinless chicken breasts, pounded to 1/4-inch thickness
» 3 cloves garlic, minced
» 1 cup dry white vermouth or dry white wine
» Juice of 1 lemon
» 1/4 cup capers
» 1/4 cup chopped fresh basil
» 1 lemon, sliced thinly into rounds

1. In a large bowl, combine flour, salt, and pepper. Dip both sides of the chicken breast in the flour mixture and place on a sheet of parchment.

2. Place olive oil in sauté pan cook chicken on one side until golden. Turn chicken and sauté other side. Add garlic in between chicken pieces.

3. When chicken is golden on both sides, add vermouth and lemon juice. Turn heat to low and add capers and basil. Add lemon slices and simmer 10 minutes.

4. Serve over a grain, such as farro or quinoa.

COOK'S TIP:
Wondra, commonly known as instant flour, is a fine granular flour that is also used to make smooth sauces. All-purpose flour can be substituted.

Exchanges/Choices
1 Starch
5 Lean Meat

Calories 295
    Calories from Fat 70
Total Fat 8.0 g
    Saturated Fat 1.7 g
    Trans Fat 0.0 g
Cholesterol 100 mg
Sodium 385 mg

Potassium 365 mg
Total Carbohydrate 14 g
    Dietary Fiber 1 g
    Sugars 1 g
Protein 38 g
Phosphorus 290 mg

Basic Grilled Chicken

SERVES: 4 / SERVING SIZE: 1/4 RECIPE

With this recipe you can create lots of great dishes like Tre Colore Salad (page 36) with Grilled Chicken, chicken salad, or serve it with any of the great side dishes in this book.

» 4 pieces boneless, skinless chicken breast (1 1/2 pounds), pounded to even thickness
» 1/4 teaspoon fine sea salt
» 1/8 teaspoon freshly ground pepper

1. Season both sides of chicken with salt and pepper. Heat grill or grill pan. Grill 3–4 minutes on each side.

COOK'S TIP:
Preheat grill or grill pan for at least 10 minutes before cooking. This will keep the chicken from sticking to the pan.

Exchanges/Choices		
5 Lean Meat		
	Calories 190	Potassium 300 mg
	Calories from Fat 35	Total Carbohydrate 0 g
	Total Fat 4.0 g	Dietary Fiber 0 g
	Saturated Fat 1.2 g	Sugars 0 g
	Trans Fat 0.0 g	Protein 36 g
	Cholesterol 100 mg	Phosphorus 265 mg
	Sodium 235 mg	

Oven-Fried Chicken

SERVES: 8 / SERVING SIZE: 1 PIECE

- » 8 chicken thighs, boned, skin removed
- » 1 16-ounce loaf rustic-style, whole-grain or whole-wheat Italian bread (such as Ciabatta)
- » 1 large clove garlic
- » 1 tablespoon Italian seasoning blend
- » 1 teaspoon fine sea salt
- » 1/2 teaspoon freshly ground black pepper
- » 1/2 cup all-purpose flour
- » 4 large eggs, whisked with 1 tablespoon water

{ COOK'S TIP:
This can be made ahead of time and frozen for reheating in a very hot oven. Defrost before reheating. }

1. Place bread, garlic, Italian seasoning blend, salt, and pepper in food processor. Process until you have large bread crumbs. This will increase the "crunch" factor.

2. Place flour in pie plate. Place eggs in another pie plate. Place bread crumbs in a third pie plate. Line a large baking sheet with parchment paper.

3. Dip chicken in flour and coat on all sides. Dip chicken in egg and then in bread crumbs. Coat evenly. Place on parchment-lined baking sheet. If you have time, refrigerate the chicken for a while before cooking time.

4. Preheat oven to 375°F. Bake chicken for 45 minutes until crispy and nicely browned. Serve with picnic condiments, salads, or applesauce.

Exchanges/Choices		
1 Starch	Calories 215	Potassium 210 mg
2 Lean Meat	Calories from Fat 70	Total Carbohydrate 16 g
1 Fat	Total Fat 8.0 g	Dietary Fiber 2 g
	Saturated Fat 2.2 g	Sugars 2 g
	Trans Fat 0.0 g	Protein 19 g
	Cholesterol 95 mg	Phosphorus 190 mg
	Sodium 330 mg	

Turkey and Sun-Dried Tomato Meatloaf or Meatballs

SERVES: 6 / SERVING SIZE: 1/6 RECIPE

I created this dish to lighten up beef meatballs and add variety to our pasta menus. Pair this with the Quick Fresh Marinara on Page 130.

» 1 1/2 cups dry bread cubes

» 1 cup dry red wine (Sangiovese or Chianti style), or chicken stock

» 1 pound ground turkey breast

» 1 cup sun-dried tomatoes (not in oil), cut in bits

» 1–2 cloves garlic, minced

» 2 shallots, minced

» 1/4 cup fresh basil, chopped, or 1 teaspoon dry basil leaves, crushed between your fingers

» 2 tablespoons fresh oregano, chopped or 1/2 teaspoon dry oregano, crushed between your fingers

» 1/4 cup pignoli nuts (pine nuts), toasted and roughly chopped

» 1/4 cup freshly grated Parmesan cheese

» 2 egg whites, or 1 whole egg

1. Preheat oven to 400°F.

2. Soak bread cubes in wine or stock.

3. Mix all ingredients together in a large bowl. Do not over mix. This will produce a tough meatloaf. Form into a loaf or meatballs and bake 45 minutes for meatloaf or 20 minutes for meatballs. (Do not use a loaf pan.)

COOK'S TIP:

Can also be made into individual meatloaves or meatballs and bake 15–20 minutes. Meatballs can be sautéed until golden.

Exchanges/Choices
1 Carbohydrate
3 Lean Meat
1/2 Fat

Calories 225
  Calories from Fat 55
Total Fat 6.0 g
  Saturated Fat 1.1 g
  Trans Fat 0.0 g
Cholesterol 50 mg
Sodium 375 mg

Potassium 615 mg
Total Carbohydrate 17 g
  Dietary Fiber 2 g
  Sugars 5 g
Protein 24 g
Phosphorus 250 mg

Enlightened Herb Roast Chicken with Garlic & Lemon

SERVES: 6 / SERVING SIZE: 1/6 RECIPE

» 1/2 cup fresh basil leaves

» 1/4 cup fresh rosemary

» 1/2 cup fresh Italian parsley

» 5–6 fresh garlic cloves, sliced into rounds

» 2 lemons, sliced thinly

» 5 pound roasting chicken

» 1 tablespoon extra virgin olive oil

» 1 teaspoon fine sea salt

» 1 teaspoon freshly ground pepper

1. Remove basil, rosemary, and parsley from their stems. Mix with garlic and lemon. Set aside.

2. Clean chicken and place it on parchment-lined baking sheet. Gently lift skin and tuck basil, parsley, and garlic until skin.

3. Lightly brush the outside of the bird with olive oil (or use mister). Sprinkle with salt and pepper. Roast chicken until golden and has reached an internal temperature of 165°F. If baking in a traditional over, cook at 400°F for 1–1 1/4 hours; for a convection oven, bake at 375°F for 50–60 minutes; if grilling, grill on medium/low with lid closed. Time will vary depending on grill. Remove and discard skin after roasting.

{ **COOK'S TIP:**
You can also use split Cornish hens, which will cook in 45 minutes, or individual chicken pieces, which will only take 20–30 minutes to cook. }

Exchanges/Choices
5 Lean Meat
1 Fat

Calories 270
  Calories from Fat 100
Total Fat 11.0 g
  Saturated Fat 2.9 g
  Trans Fat 0.0 g
Cholesterol 120 mg
Sodium 315 mg

Potassium 390 mg
Total Carbohydrate 3 g
  Dietary Fiber 1 g
  Sugars 1 g
Protein 39 g
Phosphorus 270 mg

Turkey Tenderloin with Herbs & Orange Ginger Sweet Potatoes

SERVES: 4 / SERVING SIZE: 1/4 RECIPE

Tenderloin
» 1 1/2 pounds turkey tenderloin
» 1/2 cup fresh herbs, chopped

Orange Ginger Potatoes
» 2 medium sweet potatoes
» 1 teaspoon extra virgin olive oil
» 1 (10-ounce) can mandarin oranges, drained
» 1/4 teaspoon ground ginger
» 1/4 cup chopped parsley

1. Preheat convection oven to 425°F or traditional oven to 450°F.

2. Place turkey on parchment-lined baking sheet. Coat with fresh herbs. Tuck narrow end of tenderloin under the thicker part and tie to secure. Tenderloin will cook more evenly.

3. Roast tenderloin in preheated oven until meat thermometer reaches 160°F, approximately 20 minutes. Let rest a few minutes before slicing.

4. Meanwhile, bake potatoes in microwave, about 3–4 minutes. Cut potatoes into large chunks. Place olive oil in sauté pan. Sauté potatoes, mandarin oranges, ginger, and parsley over medium heat until mixture is soft.

5. Serve orange ginger potatoes with tenderloin slices.

Exchanges/Choices		
1 Starch	Calories 275	Potassium 840 mg
5 Lean Meat	Calories from Fat 20	Total Carbohydrate 19 g
	Total Fat 2.5 g	Dietary Fiber 3 g
	Saturated Fat 0.5 g	Sugars 8 g
	Trans Fat 0.0 g	Protein 42 g
	Cholesterol 110 mg	Phosphorus 350 mg
	Sodium 100 mg	

Chicken Stuffed with Asiago, Speck & Fig

SERVES: 4 / SERVING SIZE: 1/4 RECIPE

This is an Italian-style Chicken Cordon Bleu.

» 2 tablespoons extra virgin olive oil, divided use
» 1 small onion, finely chopped
» 1 10-ounce package cremini mushrooms, half chopped and half sliced
» 2 large garlic cloves, finely minced
» 1 ounce Speck Alto Adige IGP, finely minced or purchased already chopped
» 1 6-ounce package baby spinach leaves, rinsed
» 1 cup dried figlets, cut in half
» Pinch of fine sea salt
» 2–3 grindings freshly ground black pepper
» 3 tablespoons grated Asiago Pressato DOP
» 4 boneless skinless chicken breasts (approximately 4 ounces each)
» 1/2–1 cup dry white wine (such as Orvieto, Pinot Grigio or White Vermouth)

1. In a large skillet, combine 1 tablespoon olive oil and onion. Cook over medium-high heat, approximately 3–4 minutes until onion begins to soften and becomes translucent.

2. Add the chopped mushrooms and garlic and cook another 3 minutes until mushrooms soften and start to exude liquid. Stir in Speck, spinach, and figs. Cook until spinach is almost all wilted, about 1 minute. Add salt and a few grinds of fresh black pepper. Remove from heat. Cool.

3. Add Asiago Pressato DOP (can be made a day or a few hours ahead at this point).

4. Cut a pocket in the chicken breast. Insert a long thin boning or slicing knife into the thickest side of the breast and cut a pocket. Place the stuffing into the pocket and tie with twine if desired.

(Continued on next page)

Exchanges/Choices
1 1/2 Fruit
1 Vegetable
4 Lean Meat
1 1/2 Fat

Calories 370
   Calories from Fat 115
Total Fat 13.0 g
   Saturated Fat 3.2 g
   Trans Fat 0.0 g
Cholesterol 75 mg
Sodium 315 mg

Potassium 1095 mg
Total Carbohydrate 32 g
   Dietary Fiber 5 g
   Sugars 20 g
Protein 32 g
Phosphorus 380 mg

(Chicken Stuffed with Asiago, Speck & Fig Continued)

5. Wipe out stuffing pan and add 1 tablespoon olive oil to the pan. Place chicken breast shiny side (where the skin was) down first. Brown on first side and carefully turn so you don't lose the stuffing. When browning second side, scatter sliced mushrooms on the pan surface. Brown the mushrooms with the chicken and then pour in the wine. Cover and cook 10 minutes or until internal temperature reaches 160°F.

6. Slice chicken and place on dinner plate in fan pattern. Spoon mushroom wine sauce over and serve.

} COOK'S TIP:
Can be served with Garlic Mashed Potatoes (page 123) or with Tre Colore Salad (page 36). }

Chicken Breast with Asparagus, Garlic & White Wine

SERVES: 4 / SERVING SIZE: 1/4 RECIPE

» 1/2 cup Wondra flour
» 1/2 teaspoon fine sea salt
» 1/4 teaspoon freshly ground pepper
» 4 pieces boneless, skinless chicken breast (1 1/2 pounds), pounded to even thickness
» 1 tablespoon extra virgin olive oil
» 1/2 cup white wine
» 1/2 cup low-sodium chicken stock
» 2 cloves garlic, minced
» 2 pounds fresh asparagus, trimmed
» 1/4 cup chopped fresh basil
» 1/2 cup flat Italian parsley, roughly chopped, divided use

{ **COOK'S TIP:**
To trim asparagus: hold it in both hands and bend. The ends will naturally break at the correct place. }

1. Mix flour, salt, and pepper in a shallow bowl. Dredge chicken in flour mixture.

2. Thinly film sauté pan with olive oil and heat to medium. Add chicken. Brown chicken 3–5 minutes on each side until golden.

3. Add the wine and chicken stock to deglaze pan. Add garlic and cook 2 minutes to soften. Add asparagus, basil, and 1/4 cup parsley. Cover and simmer approximately 8 minutes to ensure that chicken is cooked. (Asparagus should be lightly steamed; cooking time will vary depending on thickness of asparagus.) Garnish with remaining parsley.

4. Serve over small pasta, rice, or couscous.

Exchanges/Choices		
1 Starch	Calories 310	Potassium 635 mg
1 Vegetable	Calories from Fat 70	Total Carbohydrate 17 g
5 Lean Meat	Total Fat 8.0 g	Dietary Fiber 3 g
	Saturated Fat 1.8 g	Sugars 2 g
	Trans Fat 0.0 g	Protein 41 g
	Cholesterol 100 mg	Phosphorus 355 mg
	Sodium 410 mg	

CHAPTER 9:

Pork and Beef

The Stress Free Diabetes Kitchen

Pork and Beef

Country Pork with White Beans & Chick Peas

SERVES: 8 / SERVING SIZE: 1/8 RECIPE

I love this dish because it's easier to prepare ahead of time, it's full of healthy ingredients, it freezes well, and is also a great leftover. You could leave out the chickpeas and serve it over polenta for variety.

» 2 pounds lean, boneless country spare ribs, or pork loin cut into serving pieces
» 1 teaspoon fine sea salt with herbs
» 1/2 teaspoon freshly ground black pepper
» 2 tablespoons extra virgin olive oil
» 1 large onion, roughly chopped
» 4 garlic cloves, crushed
» 2 cups low-sodium beef broth, plus additional to thin sauce to desired consistency
» 1 cup homemade tomato sauce
» 1 15-ounce can small white beans, drained & rinsed
» 1 15-ounce can chickpeas, drained & rinsed
» 16 medium tomato slices

1. Season pork with salt and pepper.

2. Heat oil in large skillet or chef's pan. Add pork and brown on one side. Add onion and garlic. Cook until pork and onions are golden brown.

3. Add beef stock to deglaze pan. Stir to loosen browned bits. Add tomato sauce, beans, and chickpeas. Mix well. Cook a minimum of 60 minutes or longer until pork is tender. Top each serving with two tomato slices.

Exchanges/Choices
1 Starch
1 Vegetable
3 Lean Meat
1 1/2 Fat

Calories 305
  Calories from Fat 115
Total Fat 13.0 g
  Saturated Fat 3.5 g
  Trans Fat 0.0 g
Cholesterol 70 mg
Sodium 535 mg

Potassium 780 mg
Total Carbohydrate 22 g
  Dietary Fiber 7 g
  Sugars 5 g
Protein 27 g
Phosphorus 335 mg

Pork Roast Stuffed with Spinach and Prosciutto in White Wine Sauce

SERVES: 12 / SERVING SIZE: 1/12 RECIPE

This recipe is a wonderful dinner party dish that can be made ahead of time. The sauce is light and savory.

» 1 3-pound center-cut pork roast
» 1/2 teaspoon fine sea salt
» 1/2 teaspoon freshly ground black pepper
» 1 10-ounce bag baby spinach
» 4 ounces prosciutto, thinly sliced
» 1 pound fennel bulb, thinly sliced
» 1 tablespoon extra virgin olive oil
» 4 cloves garlic, minced
» 3 cups dry white Italian wine (such as Pinot Grigio or Orvieto)

1. Pound pork to an even thickness with a flat meat pounder. Sprinkle with sea salt and pepper. Top with layers of spinach, Prosciutto, and fennel. Roll tightly and tie at 2-inch intervals with twine.

2. Heat sauté pan and thinly film with extra virgin olive oil. Sear meat on all sides. Add garlic and cook until fragrant. Deglaze pan with 2 cups white wine, adding additional when needed.

3. Cover and simmer 20–30 minutes pork reaches an internal temperature of 160°F. Slice into rounds and serve with plenty of juices.

Exchanges/Choices		
3 Lean Meat	Calories 210	Potassium 560 mg
1 1/2 Fat	Calories from Fat 90	Total Carbohydrate 3 g
	Total Fat 10.0 g	Dietary Fiber 1 g
	Saturated Fat 3.4 g	Sugars 1 g
	Trans Fat 0.0 g	Protein 24 g
	Cholesterol 55 mg	Phosphorus 180 mg
	Sodium 325 mg	

Veal Barbara

This recipe is for a veal shoulder roast, not always in the meat case of your favorite store, so order ahead and they will gladly save a roast for you before it is cut into smaller pieces.

» 1 veal shoulder roast (about 3–4 pounds)
» 1 teaspoon fine sea salt
» Freshly ground black pepper
» 1 cup fresh herbs (such as basil, rosemary, chives, and parsley)
» 3–4 large cloves garlic, 1–2 minced and 1–2 chopped (keep them separate)
» 1 tablespoon extra virgin olive oil
» 1 medium onion, coarsely chopped
» 2 cups Dry Italian Red Wine (such as Barbera, Sangiovese, or Montepulciano)
» 8 ounces low-sodium beef broth

1. Preheat oven to 300°F. Lay veal roast on a parchment-lined surface. If it was tied at purchase, untie and lay flat. Pound lightly to make roast as even as possible. Sprinkle the inside of the roast with salt, a few turns of the pepper mill, and lay the herbs and garlic on the meat. Roll the meat back up and tie with string. Sprinkle with salt and pepper.

2. Coat the bottom of the pan with olive oil. Place the meat in the pan and brown on all sides. Add chopped onion and a clove or two of garlic. Sauté 1–2 minutes.

3. Deglaze the pan with 2 cups of wine. Add the beef broth and bring to a boil. Immediately turn heat off. Cover the pan and place in the oven for 1 1/2–2 hours. Cook until fork tender. Remove from oven. Let rest for a few minutes and then slice and serve with the sauce.

Exchanges/Choices	Calories 300	Potassium 540 mg
5 Lean Meat	Calories from Fat 90	Total Carbohydrate 4 g
1 Fat	Total Fat 10.0 g	Dietary Fiber 1 g
	Saturated Fat 2.4 g	Sugars 2 g
	Trans Fat 0.0 g	Protein 37 g
	Cholesterol 130 mg	Phosphorus 310 mg
	Sodium 515 mg	

Osso Buco

SERVES: 4 / SERVING SIZE: 1/4 RECIPE

Osso Buco is a classic Northern Italian dish made with veal shank and served with Risotto Milanese; however, you can also use turkey thighs or pork shanks as well. I like to serve my Osso Buco with mashed potatoes and freshly grated Asiago cheese, because it is very tasty and can be made ahead of time, as opposed to Risotto, which must be made at the last minute.

» 1/2 cup Wondra flour
» 1/2 teaspoon fine sea salt
» 1/2 teaspoon freshly ground black pepper
» 2 tablespoons extra virgin olive oil
» 4 (1–1 1/2-inch) thick slices of veal shank
» 1 cup sliced carrots
» 1 cup sliced celery
» 4 cloves garlic
» 1/2 cup chopped onion
» 1/2 cup chopped fresh basil
» 2 tablespoons chopped fresh marjoram or oregano
» 1 cup dry white wine or vermouth
» 1 cup low-sodium chicken or veal stock
» 1 15-ounce can diced tomatoes

Gremolata

» 1 lemon
» 2 cloves minced garlic
» Fresh Italian parsley

1. Place flour in large bowl or pie plate. Season with salt and pepper. Place just enough olive oil in pan to lightly coat bottom and heat. While oil is heating, dredge veal in flour. Add veal to pan and brown on both sides, approximately 5 minutes each side. Remove veal from pan.

2. Add carrots, celery, garlic, and onion. Sauté for 5 minutes and add basil and marjoram. Add wine, stock, and tomatoes. Bring to a boil. Lower heat and add veal. Cover and simmer on top of stove or in a 300°F oven for 60—90 minutes.

3. Grate zest of 1 lemon, mince 2 cloves garlic, and add 2 tablespoons parley. Mix together and reserve for garnish. This mixture is known as Gremolata.

Exchanges/Choices		
1/2 Starch	Calories 370	Potassium 935 mg
3 Vegetable	Calories from Fat 110	Total Carbohydrate 23 g
5 Lean Meat	Total Fat 12.0 g	Dietary Fiber 4 g
1 Fat	Saturated Fat 2.3 g	Sugars 7 g
	Trans Fat 0.0 g	Protein 40 g
	Cholesterol 140 mg	Phosphorus 340 mg
	Sodium 520 mg	

Grandma Ann's Meatballs

SERVES: 20/ SERVING SIZE: 1 MEATBALL

These meatballs are a Ricciardi Family Tradition, requested by the Grandchildren and enjoyed by all! While they are not just for Christmas, they were a must for the Christmas Eve Party at Grammie & Pop-Pop's.

» 3 garlic cloves, minced
» 1 small onion, minced
» 2 large eggs
» 1 tablespoon chopped fresh basil
» 1/2 cup chopped fresh parsley
» 1/4 cup freshly grated Parmesan cheese
» 1/2 teaspoon fine sea salt
» 1/2 teaspoon ground black pepper
» 1/2 cup Italian-style bread crumbs
» 1/4 cup low-sodium beef broth or red wine
» 2 pounds extra lean ground beef

1. Preheat oven to 425°F. Use a convection oven if you have it.

2. Place all ingredients, except the beef in a large bowl. Mix well. Add the beef and gently mix. Roll into desired size meatballs. (If the mixture does not hold together, add 1/4 cup additional breadcrumbs.)

3. Place the meatballs on a parchment-lined baking sheet and bake in preheated oven for 12-15 minutes to brown the outside.

4. Add to your favorite sauce or freeze until needed.

COOK'S TIP:
Mixing all the ingredients at once makes meatballs tough. This is why I mix all other ingredients first, and then add the meat.

Exchanges/Choices	Calories 85	Potassium 175 mg
2 Lean Meat	Calories from Fat 25	Total Carbohydrate 3 g
	Total Fat 3.0 g	Dietary Fiber 0 g
	Saturated Fat 1.4 g	Sugars 0 g
	Trans Fat 0.1 g	Protein 11 g
	Cholesterol 45 mg	Phosphorus 105 mg
	Sodium 150 mg	

Cotoletta Milanese

SERVES: 4 / SERVING SIZE: 1/4 RECIPE

"Scaloppini" is a very thin cut of veal, but I find that veal, pork, chicken, or turkey are all delicious prepared this way (see Cook's Tip). This dish is classically served with a mixed green salad with vinaigrette on top of the warm veal.

» 1 cup Italian seasoned bread crumbs
» 1 teaspoon of your custom herb blend or Italian Seasoning
» 1/2 teaspoon fine sea salt
» 1/2 teaspoon ground black pepper
» 2 tablespoons finely grated Parmigiano-Reggiano
» 1 large egg
» 2 egg whites
» 16 ounces scaloppini of veal, pork, chicken, or turkey
» 1 tablespoon extra virgin olive oil
» 4 cups mixed salad greens
» 4 tablespoons fat-free Italian vinaigrette

1. Mix the breadcrumbs, herb blend, salt, pepper, and cheese together in a pie plate.

2. Scramble the eggs and egg whites in a pie plate.

3. Dip the cutlets in the egg and then the bread-crumbs. You might have extra bread crumbs and egg leftover. You should discard this. The crumbs will adhere to the cutlets better if you do this and refrigerate for a few minutes or early in the day.

4. Heat the olive oil in a nonstick sauté pan and cook each cutlet until golden brown on each side. Serve with the mixed green salad and vinaigrette.

{ COOK'S TIP:
If scaloppini is not available, pound the meat to 1/4-inch thick. Place the meat between sheets of parchment and use a flat meat pounder. }

Exchanges/Choices
1/2 Starch
1/2 Carbohydrate
4 Lean Meat
1/2 Fat

Calories 275
   Calories from Fat 80
Total Fat 9.0 g
   Saturated Fat 2.4 g
   Trans Fat 0.0 g
Cholesterol 140 mg
Sodium 610 mg

Potassium 525 mg
Total Carbohydrate 15 g
   Dietary Fiber 1 g
   Sugars 2 g
Protein 31 g
Phosphorus 275 mg

Filet Mignon with Shrimp & Red Wine Reduction

SERVES: 2 / SERVING SIZE: 1/2 RECIPE

This dish makes for a lovely presentation and is really not a lot of work. It is also easy to prepare this dish for four if you're having a small dinner party.

» 2 pieces filet mignon (approximately 4 ounces each)
» 1/4 teaspoon fine sea salt
» 1/2 teaspoon freshly ground black pepper
» Few drops extra virgin olive oil

Sauce
» 1 tablespoon olive oil
» 1 large shallot, finely minced
» 1/2 cup red wine, or low-sodium broth, stock, or water can be substituted
» 1 cup beef, mushroom, or vegetable broth
» 4 jumbo shrimp, steamed, peeled, and deveined (optional)

1. Take meat out of the refrigerator 20 minutes before cooking time. Sprinkle salt and pepper on both sides of the steaks. Rub with a few drops olive oil.

2. Preheat grill pan. Cook filet for 3–5 minutes per side for rare to medium rare. (If the outside is cooking too quickly, reduce heat to medium and cover.) Test for doneness with a meat thermometer. Rare is 125°F, while medium is 140°F. Remove from pan and place on cutting board to rest.

3. In the meantime, add olive oil and shallots to small sauté pan. Cook 1 minute. Add the red wine and reduce until liquid is almost all evaporated. Add stock. Reduce by half. Serve over filet mignon.

4. Place steamed shrimp on top of the filet or serve the shrimp cocktail as an appetizer with cocktail sauce (optional).

Exchanges/Choices	Calories 265	Potassium 450 mg
4 Lean Meat	Calories from Fat 115	Total Carbohydrate 3 g
1 1/2 Fat	Total Fat 13.0 g	Dietary Fiber 1 g
	Saturated Fat 3.3 g	Sugars 1 g
	Trans Fat 0.0 g	Protein 27 g
	Cholesterol 100 mg	Phosphorus 255 mg
	Sodium 590 mg	

Pork Tenderloin with Apple Stuffing

SERVES: 10 / SERVING SIZE: 1/10 RECIPE

Pork and apples are a perfect pairing!

Apple Stuffing
- » 1 tablespoon extra virgin olive oil
- » 1 medium onion, chopped
- » 3 stalks celery, sliced
- » 1 medium apple, chopped with skin
- » 1 tablespoon poultry seasoning (such as Bell's Brand) or Italian seasoning blend
- » 1 16-ounce bag bread cubes for stuffing
- » 2–4 cups low-sodium chicken stock

2 1/2 to 3 pounds pork tenderloin

1. Thinly film the bottom of a pan with olive oil. Sauté onion, celery, and apple. Add seasoning. Sauté until fragrant. Add bread cubes and 2 cups stock. Toss well. (If moister stuffing is desired, add additional stock.) Place in shallow dish and cool before stuffing.

2. Preheat oven to 400°F for conventional oven or 375°F for convection oven.

3. Butterfly pork tenderloin. Spread with stuffing and tie. Place on parchment-lined baking sheet.

4. Roast pork tenderloin for 30 minutes. Test for doneness. A meat thermometer should read 165°F.

Exchanges/Choices
2 1/2 Starch
3 Lean Meat

Calories 325	Potassium 585 mg
Calories from Fat 55	Total Carbohydrate 39 g
Total Fat 6.0 g	Dietary Fiber 3 g
Saturated Fat 1.3 g	Sugars 5 g
Trans Fat 0.0 g	Protein 28 g
Cholesterol 60 mg	Phosphorus 275 mg
Sodium 720 mg	

Wild Boar Burger with Balsamic Tomato Condiment

SERVES: 4 / SERVING SIZE: 1/4 RECIPE

Game meats are generally very lean and add nice variety to a healthy diet. If you can afford to add a slice of cheese to your burger, an imported cheese with Truffle is a great choice.

» 1 teaspoon extra virgin olive oil
» 1 clove garlic, minced
» 14 ounces imported San Marzano Tomatoes
» 2 tablespoons Balsamic Vinegar
» 1 pound ground wild boar
» 1 tablespoon signature herb blend or Italian herb blend

1. Place olive oil in a small saucepan. Add minced garlic and cook over medium heat until fragrant. Add tomatoes and balsamic vinegar. Cook until tomatoes are reduced to the consistency of ketchup, about 15 minutes.

2. Mix boar with herb blend. Shape into four patties. Grill to desired doneness.

3. Serve on whole-grain rolls made from Whole-Wheat Pizza Dough recipe (page 142). The Oven Baked Herb Onion Rings (page 27) are also a nice compliment.

Exchanges/Choices		
1 Vegetable	Calories 175	Potassium 540 mg
3 Lean Meat	Calories from Fat 45	Total Carbohydrate 6 g
	Total Fat 5.0 g	Dietary Fiber 1 g
	Saturated Fat 1.3 g	Sugars 3 g
	Trans Fat 0.0 g	Protein 25 g
	Cholesterol 65 mg	Phosphorus 135 mg
	Sodium 195 mg	

Asian Pork & Bok Choy "Lasagna"

SERVES: 4 / SERVING SIZE: 1/4 RECIPE

This low carb Asian-inspired dish is so easy to make and adds something a little different to your repertoire. Use the leftover Bok Choy to add to other dishes during the week, such as stir-fry, salads, or soups.

» 1 pound (96% lean) ground pork
» 1/2 cup dry white wine (such as Orvieto, Pinot Grigio, or Sauvignon Blanc)
» 1 bunch (about 2 cups) Bok Choy, washed, trimmed, and diced (white part only)
» 1 bunch scallions (green onions), washed, trimmed, and cut into 1/2-inch thick strips
» 1 11-ounce can Mandarin oranges, drained (reserve liquid)
» 2–3 tablespoons chili garlic paste
» 1 tablespoon light soy sauce

1. Heat large nonstick sauté pan and brown pork. Deglaze pan with the wine. Add diced Bok Choy and scallions. Stir fry to soften the vegetables, approximately 3 minutes. Add the juice from the oranges, the chili garlic paste, and soy sauce. Stir well to blend and heat to a boil. Turn heat off.

2. Place large Bok Choy leaves in bottom of 8 × 8-inch square baking dish so that they cover the bottom. Spread half of the pork mixture on top. Add another layer of Bok Choy leaves. Repeat with remaining pork mixture. Top with more Bok Choy leaves. Sprinkle the oranges over all.

3. Cover with plastic wrap and place in microwave on high 3-4 minutes to wilt the top Bok Choy leaves. Let rest 1 minute and serve.

Exchanges/Choices
1/2 Fruit
1 Vegetable
4 Lean Meat

Calories 215
 Calories from Fat 45
Total Fat 5.0 g
 Saturated Fat 1.7 g
 Trans Fat 0.0 g
Cholesterol 65 mg
Sodium 365 mg

Potassium 915 mg
Total Carbohydrate 14 g
 Dietary Fiber 3 g
 Sugars 9 g
Protein 28 g
Phosphorus 280 mg

Chipotle Skirt Steak

SERVES: 4 / SERVING SIZE: 1/4 RECIPE

Skirt steak is a very lean cut of beef that is found on the inside of the ribs. It is very thin and cooks very quickly and is great when cooked on a grill pan.

» 1/2 cup panko
» 1 tablespoon crushed chipotle pepper
» 1 pound skirt steak
» 1 tablespoon extra virgin olive oil

1. Mix the panko and the chipotle pepper in a small bowl.

2. Coat the steak with the olive oil. Dip in the seasoned panko.

3. Grill 3 minutes on first side. Turn and grill second side until steak is medium (See Cook's Tip). This will vary based on the thickness of the skirt steak.

4. Slice across the grain and serve with a cherry tomato and parsley salad. You can also make this salad with cilantro instead of parsley to compliment the chipotle.

Exchanges/Choices
1/2 Starch
3 Lean Meat
1 1/2 Fat

Calories 245
　Calories from Fat 115
Total Fat 13.0 g
　Saturated Fat 4.0 g
　Trans Fat 0.0 g
Cholesterol 75 mg
Sodium 80 mg

Potassium 285 mg
Total Carbohydrate 6 g
　Dietary Fiber 0 g
　Sugars 1 g
Protein 25 g
Phosphorus 220 mg

CHAPTER 10:
Desserts

The Stress Free Diabetes Kitchen

Cannoli Cups

SERVES: 6 / SERVING SIZE: 1/6 RECIPE

Here is a great alternative to the higher fat Cannoli with its fried shell.

» 4 sheets (14 × 9-inch) phyllo,
» olive oil spray
» 1 cup low-fat ricotta cheese
» 1 teaspoon vanilla
» 1 teaspoon Grand Marnier, or any orange flavored liquor
» 1/2 teaspoon ground cinnamon
» 1 tablespoon Confectioner's sugar
» 1/4-ounce piece of chocolate
» 2 tablespoons chopped nuts (such as pistachio or walnuts)

1. Preheat oven to 350°F.

2. Lay one sheet of phyllo on parchment-lined cutting board. Spray with olive oil spray. Repeat with all four sheets. Cut into six equal size squares. Place each square in a muffin or cupcake pan. Bake 5–6 minutes or until golden brown.

3. Mix remaining ingredients together. Just before serving, fill each of the Phyllo cups with equal portions of the cheese mixture. Garnish with shaved chocolate and crushed nuts.

{ COOK'S TIP:
» Use a fine cheese grater for the chocolate.
» Phyllo dough is available frozen and should be defrosted in the refrigerator, not in the microwave. }

Exchanges/Choices		
1/2 Carbohydrate	Calories 95	Potassium 95 mg
1 Lean Meat	Calories from Fat 35	Total Carbohydrate 10 g
1/2 Fat	Total Fat 4.0 g	Dietary Fiber 1 g
	Saturated Fat 1.8 g	Sugars 4 g
	Trans Fat 0.0 g	Protein 6 g
	Cholesterol 15 mg	Phosphorus 95 mg
	Sodium130 mg	

Lemon Chiffon with Fresh Berries

SERVES: 6 / SERVING SIZE: 1/2 CUP

This deliciously sweet tart dessert is very refreshing with a melt in your mouth quality; it is light enough to enjoy without feeling guilty. You can make it a day or two before a party and it will be even better.

» 1/3 cup fresh lemon juice, strained of seeds (about 2 large lemons)
» 1/2 cup granulated sugar or Splenda
» 4 large eggs
» 3 cups fresh berries (such as strawberries, blueberries, and blackberries)

{ COOK'S TIP:
Lemon Chiffon also makes a very nice dip for a fruit platter. Serve it in a bowl over ice to keep it chilled. }

1. Place lemon juice and sugar in saucepan. Heat and stir until sugar dissolves. Remove from heat.

2. Crack eggs into the bowl and whisk well. Slowly pour the lemon sugar mix into the eggs while whisking. Whisk for 1 minute and then return the egg mixture to the saucepan. Whisk and cook on low to medium for several minutes, until the egg mixture thickens. (The more you whisk, the lighter the mixture will be.) This will take 2–5 minutes depending on your equipment. When it coats the back of a spoon it is ready to be removed from the heat and refrigerated. (It will thicken more as it cools.) Cool one hour or more.

3. Place some of the lemon chiffon in a dessert glass or bowl and spoon berries over or layer lemon cream and berries. Top with berries.

Exchanges/Choices		
2 Carbohydrate	Calories 145	Potassium 155 mg
1/2 Fat	Calories from Fat 30	Total Carbohydrate 26 g
	Total Fat 3.5 g	Dietary Fiber 2 g
	Saturated Fat 1.1 g	Sugars 22 g
	Trans Fat 0.0 g	Protein 5 g
	Cholesterol 125 mg	Phosphorus 80 mg
	Sodium 50 mg	

Fresh Picked Apple Crunch Cake

SERVES: 16 / SERVING SIZE: 1/16 RECIPE

This cake is great for a brunch or dessert.

- » 2 cups plain, low-fat yogurt
- » 2 eggs or 4 egg whites
- » 1 teaspoon vanilla
- » 2 cups all-purpose flour
- » 3/4 cup Splenda
- » 1 teaspoon baking powder
- » 1 teaspoon baking soda
- » 1/2 teaspoon fine sea salt
- » 1 cup walnuts, chopped
- » 1 teaspoon cinnamon
- » 2 cups unpeeled and chopped baking apples (Macintosh, Winesap, Rome, Empire, or Granny Smith)
- » Nonstick cooking spray

1. In a large bowl, mix yogurt, eggs, and vanilla.

2. In another large bowl, mix flour, Splenda, baking powder, baking soda, salt, walnuts, and cinnamon. Add apples and mix.

3. Combine wet and dry ingredients, mixing just until moistened.

4. Spray a 10-inch tube pan or spring form pan with nonstick cooking spray. Pour batter into pan.

5. Bake at 350°F for 50–60 minutes. Sprinkle top with cinnamon and sugar mixture, if desired.

{ COOK'S TIP:
This is a very moist cake and should be refrigerated after a day because of the active cultures of the yogurt. }

Exchanges/Choices
1 1/2 Carbohydrate
1 Fat

Calories 145
    Calories from Fat 55
Total Fat 6.0 g
    Saturated Fat 1.0 g
    Trans Fat 0.0 g
Cholesterol 20 mg
Sodium 205 mg

Potassium 145 mg
Total Carbohydrate 19 g
    Dietary Fiber 1 g
    Sugars 5 g
Protein 5 g
Phosphorus 130 mg

Prosecco Poached Pears with Caramel

SERVES: 8 / SERVING SIZE: 1/2 PEAR

» 4 Bosc pears
» 1 bottle of Prosecco (Italian sparkling
   wine from the Veneto)
» 6–8 whole cloves
» 1 teaspoon ground cinnamon
» 1/2 teaspoon vanilla
» 7 ounces sweetened condensed milk

{ **COOK'S TIP:**
Leftover caramel sauce can be
refrigerated and microwaved
to reuse. }

1. Peel the pears and cut a little slice off the bottom so that they stand upright. Leave stems on.

2. Place pears, Prosecco, cloves, cinnamon, and vanilla in a saucepan that holds the pears snuggly. (The liquid should come up to the top of the pears.)

3. Bring to a boil, lower heat, and simmer for 20–30 minutes, until the pears are fork tender. Cool in the poaching liquid.

4. In the meantime, place the condensed milk in a small saucepan and bring to a boil. Immediately turn down to low and cook and stir until the milk thickens and becomes a slightly darker caramel color

5. Serve the pears in a puddle of the caramel and drizzle some of the caramel over the pear.

Exchanges/Choices		
2 Carbohydrate	Calories 160	Potassium 230 mg
1/2 Fat	Calories from Fat 25	Total Carbohydrate 32 g
	Total Fat 3.0 g	Dietary Fiber 3 g
	Saturated Fat 1.8 g	Sugars 27 g
	Trans Fat 0.0 g	Protein 3 g
	Cholesterol 10 mg	Phosphorus 95 mg
	Sodium 45 mg	

Citrus Cake

SERVES: 12/ SERVING SIZE: 1/12 RECIPE

This is a light, simple, yet delicious cake that you can proudly serve. It is also lovely garnished with fresh fruit.

- » 1 cup Splenda
- » 1/4 cup canola oil
- » 2 tablespoons lemon or orange zest
- » Juice of 1 lemon or orange
- » 2 eggs, lightly beaten
- » 1 cup plain nonfat yogurt (or lemon yogurt)
- » 2 cups all-purpose flour
- » 1 tablespoon baking powder
- » Nonstick cooking spray

COOK'S TIP:
This also works well in a cakelette or cupcake pan. For cakelettes or cupcakes, pour batter in pan and fill 3/4 full. Bake 30 minutes.

1. Preheat oven to 350°F.

2. In a large mixing bowl, combine Splenda, oil, zest, and juice. Add the eggs and mix completely. Add yogurt.

3. Combine flour and baking powder. Slowly add mixing bowl until well blended.

4. Lightly spray bundt pan with nonstick cooking spray. Bake 50 minutes or until toothpick comes out clean (cake pan sizes vary so test carefully and adjust baking time accordingly).

5. Sprinkle with Confectioners Sugar and garnish with edible flowers, if desired.

Exchanges/Choices		
1 1/2 Carbohydrate	Calories 150	Potassium 85 mg
1 Fat	Calories from Fat 55	Total Carbohydrate 20 g
	Total Fat 6.0 g	Dietary Fiber 1 g
	Saturated Fat 0.7 g	Sugars 4 g
	Trans Fat 0.0 g	Protein 4 g
	Cholesterol 30 mg	Phosphorus 185 mg
	Sodium 115 mg	

Index

The Stress Free Diabetes Kitchen

Alphabetical Index

Subject Index